CANCER AND HEART DISEASE

MICHIO KUSHI

CANCER AND HEART DISEASE

The Macrobiotic Approach to Degenerative Disorders

with

Robert S. Mendelsohn, M.D., *former Chairman, Medical Licensure Committee, State of Illionois; Author of* Confessions of a Medical Heretic

William Castelli, M.D., *Medical Director, Framingham Heart Study; Lecturer on Preventive Medicine and Epidemiology, Harvard Medical School*

Paul Schulman, *former Director, Lemuel Shattuck Hospital, Boston; Assistant Professor of Community Health, Tufts School of Medicine*

Keith Block, M.D., *Medical/Nutritional Consultant, CBS Radio, Chicago*

Richard Donze, D.O., *Family Medicine Clinic, Methodist Hospital, Philadelphia*

Lawrence H. Kushi, *Researcher, Department of Nutrition, Harvard School of Public Health*

Frank Kern, *Assistant Director, Tidewater Detention Center, Virginia Beach*

Christiane Northrup, M.D., *Fellow of the American College of Obstetricians and Gynecologists*

William Tara, *Director, Kushi Institute, Boston*

Edited by **Edward Esko**

Japan Publications, Inc.

Published by JAPAN PUBLICATIONS, INC., Tokyo

Distributors:
UNITED STATES: *Kodansha International/USA, Ltd., through Harper & Row, Publishers, Inc., 10 East 53rd Street, New York, New York 10022.* SOUTH AMERICA: *Harper & Row, Publishers, Inc., International Department.* CANADA: *Fitzhenry & Whiteside Ltd., 150 Lesmill Road, Don Mills, Ontario M3B 2T6.* MEXICO AND CENTRAL AMERICA: *HARLA S. A. de C. V. Apartado 30–546, Mexico 4, D. F.* BRITISH ISLES: *International Book Distributors Ltd., 66 Wood Lane End, Hemel Hempstead, Herts HP2 4RG.* EUROPEAN CONTINENT: *Boxerbooks, Inc., Limmatstrasse 111, 8031 Zurich.* AUSTRALIA AND NEW ZEALAND: *Book Wise (Australia) Pty. Ltd., 104–8 Sussex Street, Sydney 2000.* THE FAR EAST AND JAPAN: *Japan Publications Trading Co., Ltd., 1–2–1, Sarugaku-cho, Chiyoda-ku, Tokyo 101.*

First edition: November 1982

LCCC No. 82–81053
ISBN 0–87040–515–2

Printed in U.S.A.

Foreword

When I first started to recognize the importance of health, I was studying and pursuing the possibility of establishing a world federation during the years following the Second World War. As my study deepened, I realized that the problem of individual health is directly related to the most fundamental questions of life: "Where have we come from?" "How have we come to appear on this earth?" and "Where do we go to in the future?" Hence I also began to search for the secret of life while seeking solutions to the problems of physical and psychological disorders

Since the dawn of history, the human intellect has continually sought for a solution to the problems of sickness, proverty, war, misery, and conflict and striven for some practical means to overcome suffering as a foundation for enduring peace. The magnitude of the problems confronting us today requires that we completely review and reevaluate our entire way of thinking according to the proper understanding of humanity's origin and destiny. It also may be necessary to set a new direction for the course of civilization itself.

My search for a solution to these problems has continually been inspired by the immortal vision of one peaceful world. I soon realized that in order to succeed, I had to discover a practical method to enable people to recover from the degenerative conditions which now affect society. The problems of cancer and heart disease, together with psychological and mental disorders which prevail today, are in many ways symbolic of the overall trend which threatens the entire world in this latter part of the twentieth century.

In my view, cancer, heart disease, and other physical disorders are a direct result of a lack of understanding of what humanity is, together with a confused view of life, nature, and the universe. If we are able to discover the principles which govern the natural world—of which we are a part—and apply these principles to develop the proper way of life for humanity on this planet, a direct solution for the current crisis of biological degeneration will have been found. In order for this solution to be fundamental and long-lasting, these principles must be applied not only in the biological realm, but also in the psychological, social, philosophical, and spiritual dimensions.

After many years of observation and experience, I have discovered that human life in all its dimensions is nothing but the result of the interrelationship between food and the surrounding environment. The natural environment includes the multitude of factors which make up the universal background of life, such as cosmic influences, celestial radiation, galactic and solar forces, planetary movements —including those of the Earth—and atmospheric conditions which vary according to altitude, season, and geographical location. Also included are the various influences on our thinking and behavior which are created by our human environment, civilization. Similarly, *food* includes all of the factors that we consume or take in from the environment both in the form of vibrational forces such as light, sound, and electromagnetic radiation, together with the biological, biochemical, and chemical factors that we eat, drink, and breathe.

Because we are able to exercise control over what we eat and drink, physical food is the most important environmental influence in determining our individual health and happiness. Our ability to control the other environmental factors that we take in is much more limited in comparison to the freedom that we exercise in regard to our daily food. Control over our daily dietary practice is the key to solving all physical, psychological, and social problems.

The differences in dietary practice among people, together with variations in their natural and social environments, cause some to develop and suffer from physical or psychological ailments and others to remain free of disorders. These differences also produce the tremendous variation in cultural patterns and ways of thinking which exist throughout the world.

During the period from 1960–65, I began a serious study of degenerative diseases, especially cancer. As a part of this study, I examined many of the current scientific theories regarding the cause of cancer, including those which stated that the disease was hereditary, or that it resulted from exposure to environmental pollutants and radiation, or that it was caused by viruses, microorganisms, or various psychological or psychosomatic factors. However, reviewing the medical research, I felt as if I were wandering in a dark jungle with no escape. Therefore, I decided to detach myself from these limited approaches and change my orientation from a *microbiotic* to a *macrobiotic* view. I began by reviewing the understanding of the order of the universe and its law of change from the sub-atomic to the galactic levels. From this perspective, I studied the rise and fall of societies and reexamined the phenomenon of biological degeneration in relation to dietary and environmental influences.

It soon became clear that like all degenerative diseases, cancer is primarily the result of a daily diet and way of life which are not in harmony with the surrounding environment. Practically speaking, the incidences of cancer, heart disease, and various other degenerative disorders have continued to increase as people have shifted from the more balanced traditional dietary pattern based around whole cereal grains, organically grown fresh vegetables and fruits, beans and sea vegetables, and other regional products toward the modern dietary pattern based on an increased consumption of meat and dairy products, fatty and oily foods, and overly refined, chemicalized, industrialized, and artificial food items. The increase in physical and psychological degeneration which we are experiencing is due primarily to the changing dietary patterns of modern civilization.

Among the many varieties of disease, two apparently opposite categories of causes and symptoms stand out. For example, among circulatory disorders there are those which involve an overexpansion of the heart and blood vessels, leading to low blood pressure and those in which the circulatory vessels are overly contracted, leading to high blood pressure. Similarly, there are two apparently opposite categories of cancer; those which appear more toward the skin and peripheral regions of the body, such as skin and breast cancer and those which appear in the internal organs or in the depths of the body, such as liver or pancreatic cancer. No matter how complicated the symptoms may appear, all sicknesses can be understood in terms of these two apparently different tendencies. Needless to say, a countless variety of symptoms exist as gradations between these two apparently opposite tendencies.

The solution for heart disease, cancer, and all other degenerative diseases, including diabetes, arthritis, epilepsy, polio, cerebral palsy, physical and mental retardation, and schizophrenia, paranoia, and other psychological disturbances can be found in various modifications of a way of eating in which these two opposite tendencies are brought into a more moderate balance. The traditional diet of humanity protected against degenerative diseases for thousands of years. The Standard Macrobiotic Diet is based on these principles and consists of the following food groups:

1. 50%–60% whole cereal grains and their products;
2. 5%–10% (one or two cups or small bowls) of soup, with land and sea vegetables as the main ingredients;
3. 20%–30% locally available vegetables, the majority of which are cooked;
4. 5%–10% beans and sea vegetables, as sources of high-quality protein and minerals.

In addition, these foods may be occasionally supplemented, if desired, with fish and seafood, locally available fruits in season, seeds and nuts, various nonaromatic and nonstimulant seasonings and condiments, and nonfragrant, nonaromatic grain and herbal beverages.

Of course, this standard dietary approach requires modification for each person or illness, depending upon the particular condition and symptoms. For example, in some cases, particular varieties of grains and vegetables may need to be emphasized over others, certain methods of cooking and preparation may be preferred, or particular supplementary foods may need to be included while others may need to be avoided.

Over the last twenty years, many thousands of people from all over the world have recovered from numerous disorders through this macrobiotic dietary approach. Another remarkable fact in many of these cases has been the development of a more peaceful and serene mental condition, along with the establishment of more satisfying family relationships based on admiration and respect for elders and love and care toward children and younger associates. Many of these people have also developed a sense of aesthetic appreciation, along with a profound sense of wonder and gratitude toward nature and other people.

As many of these experiences confirm, the recovery of physical health often leads to a subtle but profound change in the entire personality, including the development of more satisfying human relations and a deep appreciation for life on all levels. It is through changes such as these that a peaceful solidarity can develop within society, leading eventually to a peaceful world community. I am firmly convinced that this simple, practical, and effective approach, which can be applied by anyone in daily life, offers a definite solution for the problem of degenerative sickness, as well as for the various struggles, difficulties, and conflicts in society.

In this book, which is based on materials compiled from articles, speeches, and case-studies over the last six years, the basic applications of the marcobiotic way of life are presented, especially as they apply to the problem of degenerative illness. On behalf of our many macrobiotic friends and associates throughout the world, I wish to express my gratitude to all of the contributors to this book for sharing the endless dream of a healthy, peaceful, and productive society and for their efforts to improve the health and well-being of all people. By offering such continual inspiration and enlightenment to society, these associates are contributing to the realization of a new dimension of civilization based on a more healthy and constructive direction. I also wish to thank Edward Esko, who has studied various issues related to the recovery of humanity with me for the past ten years, for editing this book and, on behalf of all of the contributors, extend my gratitude to the publisher, Japan Publications, Inc.

Furthermore, this dream of establishing a healthy and peaceful society through a more natural and macrobiotic way of life is now being shared by some millions of people throughout the world. Further information about the macrobiotic way of life, including educational programs and cooking classes, can be obtained from the Kushi Foundation, the Kushi Institute, the East West Foundation, or the *East West Journal*, all of which can be contacted at P.O. Box 1100, Brookline Village, MA 02147. Information can also be obtained from more than 300 East West and Macrobiotic Centers throughout North America, Europe, Central and South America, the Middle East, India, Southeast Asia, Australia, and the Far East.

MICHIO KUSHI
Brookline, Massachusetts
July, 1982

Contents

Introduction

Cancer and heart disease are problems which affect everyone in modern society. Either through personal experience or through that of family members or friends, an increasing number of people are confronting these disorders.

For more than thirty years, Michio Kushi and his associates throughout the world have recommended a natural, macrobiotic approach to these and other illnesses. Through his lectures, conferences, and educational activities, Mr. Kushi has guided hundreds of thousands of people in establishing health and well-being for themselves and their families. At the same time, his association with leaders in the medical, scientific, and research fields has contributed greatly toward the new model of health care and social rehabilitation that is beginning to emerge.

In the area of food distribution, Mr. Kushi and associates helped pioneer of the natural foods movement through their efforts over the past fifteen years in developing Erewhon, a company which has consistently maintained the highest standards of quality within the natural foods industry. At the same time, the *East West Journal*, which was started by Mr. Kushi's students, has continuously inspired the worldwide movement toward better nutrition, natural and macrobiotic approaches to health care, natural farming, and a sound and healthful approach to living.

Ten years ago, Mr. Kushi and associates in Boston established the East West Foundation. I had the privilege to participate in the development of many of the Foundation's educational programs during the 1970s, including annual residential seminars at Amherst and Pine Manor Colleges; Kushi International Seminars throughout Europe, South America, and the Far East; annual medical conferences and public symposia on the macrobiotic approach to cancer and other disorders; and the establishment of regional educational centers throughout the United States and Canada.

In 1978, Mr. Kushi and associates established teacher training centers in London, Amsterdam, and Boston, under the name of the Kushi Institute. Since then more than 2,000 people have participated in Institute programs, and many Institute graduates are now making positive contributions to society through their educational and other activities.

Over the past ten years, institutions such as the Harvard Medical School and Tufts Nutrition Center in Boston have contacted Mr. Kushi for the purpose of conducting research on the macrobiotic way of eating. In 1973, a team of Harvard researchers began studying the effects of the macrobiotic diet on the major risk factors associated with heart disease. Encouraged by promising results, Frank Sacks, M.D., William Castelli, M.D., and associates are planning additional research which could demonstrate that the macrobiotic diet is effective in reversing cardiovascular disease. One project currently being considered involves the introduction of the macrobiotic diet to a group of patients with atherosclerosis, or deposits of fat and cholesterol in the arteries around the heart.

In 1981, a non-profit organization, the Kushi Foundation, was established to assist in the coordination of these educational and research activities. Over the next several years, the Foundation plans to begin compiling case histories and statistical data on many thousands of people who are practicing macrobiotics, as a valuable resource for future studies on the relationship between diet and health.

Many physicians throughout the world have attended Mr. Kushi's seminars and are now incorporating macrobiotic methods in the care of a wide variety of illnesses. In the United States, Keith Block, M.D., an associate of Dr. Robert S. Mendelsohn, is compiling data on a number of patients in the Chicago area who are utilizing the macrobiotic approach, while in Philadelphia, Dr. Richard Donze is compiling similiar data at the Family Medicine Clinic at the Methodist Hospital. At the same time, institutions such as the Lemuel Shattuck Hospital in Boston and the Methodist Hospital in Philadelphia have begun highly successful macrobiotic meal services for their staffs. The Shattuck Hospital has also begun to offer the macrobiotic diet to a group of elderly mental patients as a part of an ongoing research program.

To help meet the growing need for qualified macrobiotic cooks and cooking instructors for home service, private classes, and institutional needs, the Kushi Institute Cook Referral Service was started in 1981. The CRS provides cooks and instructors trained in the principles and art of macrobiotic cooking, primarily for individuals and families who are interested in learning the fundamentals of macrobiotic food preparation. CRS members are qualified to prepare delicious and wholesome meals and through teaching and assistance, to instruct clients in proper cooking techniques.

Several projects have also been established in the area of social rehabilitation, including a highly successful program in Portugal in which macrobiotic food is being made available to a group of inmates within a maximum security prison, and a preliminary research project at the Tidewater Detention Home near Virginia Beach, Virginia on the relationship between refined sugar consumption and asocial behavior. The results of the Tidewater project have encouraged Department of Corrections officials to approve a plan to begin a macrobiotic meal service at the center in order to study the effects of a well balanced, whole foods diet on behavior.

In his other Japan Publications titles*, Michio Kushi has introduced the principles of macrobiotics, illustrating their application in a variety of domains. In this, his latest volume, he concentrates on the macrobiotic approach to the prevention of and potential for recovering from degenerative illnesses, especially cancer and heart disease. He is assisted in this effort by a number of associates, all of whom are pioneering new approaches in the fields of health care, medical research, social rehabilitation, and macrobiotic education.

Along with a readily adaptable, common sense approach to food and cooking,

---

* See Bibliography.

macrobiotics offers a holistic view of illnesses such as cancer and heart disease. Therefore, according to the macrobiotic view:

1. Cancer is seen as a total illness involving an organism as a whole, and not as an isolated cellular disorder;
2. A tumor is understood to be the focal point for the localization of toxic excess which has accumulated in the organism;
3. Although seemingly antagonistic, a tumor is viewed as serving the beneficial function of removing toxins from general circulation, thereby allowing the organism as a whole to continue functioning;
4. Cancer is seen as a degenerative process which is rooted in the quality of the daily foods, beverages, and other environmental factors which are constantly being taken in;
5. This process is understood to be nourished by the excessive intake of foods and beverages which are either extremely yin (expansive) or extremely yang (constrictive); or by the excessive intake of both extremes. More yin cancers have a tendency to appear in the upper or more peripheral regions of the body, while more yang cancers tend to appear lower and more deep within the body;
6. This process is understood to be potentially reversible through a change in the quality of the foods, beverages, and other environmental factors which produce and nourish it;
7. No two cancers are identical; each is understood to arise from a unique set of environmental and dietary circumstances.

In the opening chapter, Mr. Kushi explains the macrobiotic view and also discusses the present crisis of biological degeneration which threatens the continuation of society. He then compares the macrobiotic view of cancer with modern theories about the disease, discussing its cause, mechanism, and process of development; and introduces several traditional methods for diagnosing the disease; and then cites the factors involved in the recovery from cancer. Here he presents the Standard Macrobiotic Diet, outlining a variety of modifications for individual circumstances based on the classification of cancer types according to the traditional perspective of yin and yang. This section includes guidelines for preparation and use of special dishes, macrobiotic condiments, and external applications, and a variety of recommendations for a healthful, natural life-style.

In his discussion of heart disease, Mr. Kushi introduces the classification of cardiovascular disorders according to yin and yang with specific dietary adjustments presented for each type. A variety of special dishes are introduced, many of which have been traditionally used for thousands of years. Several unique methods for diagnosing heart conditions are also presented in this section.

In the concluding section, Mr. Kushi discusses the implications of a recent computer study on possible medically related future trends, particularly the present direction toward automation of the human organism. He concludes by contrasting the natural, macrobiotic approach to maintaining health with the rapidly developing trend toward more artificial and technological approaches to sickness.

In the second chapter, two leading holistic physicians, Christiane Northrup,

M.D. and Keith Block, M.D., present their view of the cancer problem, with
emphasis on holistic and dietary approaches. In the following chapter, William
Castelli, M.D., Medical Director of the Framingham Heart Study, and Lawrence
H. Kushi, of the Department of Nutrition at the Harvard School of Public
Health, detail the epidemiological links and other evidence of the relationship
between diet and heart disease. A summary of the macrobiotic/cardiovascular
research conducted by the Harvard School of Medicine is also presented, as is a
discussion of how the Standard Macrobiotic Diet fulfills, and in some cases
surpasses, the recommendations set forth in *Dietary Goals for the United States.*

We have also included a section of statements from this landmark document
issued five years ago by the Senate Nutrition Committee.

The next chapter, *Macrobiotics, Preventive Medicine, and Society*, includes
statements by Robert S. Mendelsohn, M.D., the well-known medical author and
syndicated columnist, on recent developments pointing to a reorientation of
priorities in modern medical practice; Paul Schulman, former Director of the
Shattuck Hospital, on the contribution of macrobiotics to the dynamic new model
of health care which is now emerging; Richard Donze, D.O., on the shortcomings
of the "crisis management" approach to disease, and the need for meaningful
approaches to prevention; Frank Kern, Assistant Director of the Tidewater
Detention Home in Virginia on the relationship between diet and behavior,
and the need for a more fundamental approach to criminal rehabilitation; Kristen
Schmidt, a registered nurse, on the integration of macrobiotic methods in the
care of patients; and William Tara, the Educational Director of the Kushi Institute
in Boston, on the social implications of prevention.

The final chapter includes three sections of case histories dealing with cancer
and cancer related sicknesses; with cardiovascular disorders; and with miscel-
laneous illnesses. Also included is a report by Hideo Ohmori of the Japan Macrobiotic Association on his experiences over the past twenty years in use of the
macrobiotic approach for a variety of disorders, including cancer and sicknesses
resulting from exposure to atomic radiation; and a report by Norman Ralston,
D.V.M., on the use of the macrobiotic diet in his veterinary practice in Dallas,
Texas.

The Appendixes at the end of the Chapters include a listing of macrobiotic
external applications and natural remedies with instructions for their preparation;
a summary of the evidence linking diet with cancer and heart disease; and a history
and overview of the macrobiotic food program at the Shattuck Hospital written
by Thomas Igelhart and Eric Zutrau, both of whom were responsible for initiating
the program. The appeneixes at the back of the book include the *Food Policy
Recommendations for the United States* presented five years ago by Mr. Kushi
and associates at the White House, and a summary of East West Foundation
activities in the diet and health area.

This volume, then, serves as an introduction for medical and health professionals to the applications of the macrobiotic approach and to its growing significance in the context of the changing world of medicine and health care. It also
serves as an introductory guide for the individual reader to the understanding and

practical application of this approach in daily life.

I would like to express appreciation to all of the people who have contributed to the creation of this book. The origins of this present volume date back to 1976, when, under Mr. Kushi's guidance, the East West Foundation began to compile case histories and other materials on the macrobiotic approach to cancer. I wish to thank all of the people who assisted with the preparation, publication and distribution of these materials in *Cancer and Diet, the Cancer Prevention Diet*, and other Foundation reports. I also thank all of the people who helped arrange the annual Conferences on the Macrobiotic Approach to Cancer and Degenerative Illnesses from 1977–1981, along with all of those who spoke at these gatherings, including Michio Kushi, Robert S. Mendelsohn, M.D., William Castelli, M.D., and many of the other contributors to this book. I would also like to thank Peter Harris for contributing the illustrations for this book, and the contributors who wrote articles or case histories especially for publication in this new volume. I also thank Dr. Block and Dr. Northrup for their careful reviewing of the case histories contained in this volume; John Mann and Meg Seaker for their editorial comments and assistance; and Diane Coffey and others for assisting with the final preparation of the text.

EDWARD ESKO
Brookline, Massachusetts
July, 1982

Chapter 1

The Macrobiotic Approach

Michio Kushi

During the sixteenth century, Western countries spread their influence from Europe to the entire world, including all of Asia. From then on, a universal wind of science and technology began to blow throughout the world. It took a long time, nearly 400 years, before the people of Asia could assimilate and understand Western methods of expression, along with Western technology and science and, by learning this way of expressing themselves, begin to present their universal, traditional philosophy and way of life in terms that all people could understand.

A new era is now beginning, through the combination and synthesis of East and West. Previous distinctions between the Occident and the Orient are no longer applicable. In many ways, all people on the earth have become one, sharing the same level of culture and civilization, the same means of communication and transportation, and a similar manner of eating and living. At the present time, all people of the world also share the same destiny.

At present, we all face the greatest crisis in the history of the human race, regardless of our nationality, religion, or cultural background. This crisis is the result of nothing less than the complete and all-pervasive degeneration of mankind on all levels—physical, psychological, social, and spiritual. We, modern homo sapiens, are rapidly degenerating because we have ignored, especially during the past half century, the order of nature, the order of the universe, of you may say the law of God. Instead, our civilization has developed with the primary motivation of profit-making or commercialism. Modern economic systems have been organized largely with this goal in mind, without genuinely considering what would serve for the health and well-being of our society.

We have now come to the verge of witnessing the collapse of our entire modern civilization. If we do not turn our direction soon, by the year 2000, which is less than twenty years away, 50 percent or more of the people in the United States will constantly suffer from some type of degenerative disease, including cancer, heart disease, psychological disorders, diabetes, and a most of others. At the same time, the other half of the population will have to work to support them, while everyone will be forced to bear the tremendous cost of health care, social security, welfare, and insurance. If we continue in this direction, it is inevitable that in another ten to twenty years, the United States will collapse.

Fifteen years ago, I met with a group of doctors at a major New York hospital. When they asked my opinion about the cause of cancer, I simply stated, "Diet." They asked if I thought that hereditary and environmental factors were also important, and I replied, "Those are relatively minor; diet is the main problem." They looked at each other and shrugged their shoulders. After several moments of silence, one of the doctors finally said, "Can you demonstrate whether diet is the main factor or not?" I replied, "Yes, if you give me several of your patients. I will leave my address and telephone number. Please contact me anytime." I never heard from them again.

Several years ago, during a luncheon with a group of professors and scientists from a Boston area university, we began to discuss a number of health issues, especially the continual increase in cancer and heart disease. I mentioned that in order to reverse this trend, it would be necessary for most people to change their diet and life-style. Otherwise, the future of mankind was very dark. Upon hearing my remark, they started to argue among themselves, saying things like, "Are we really degenerating, or are we in the process of development?" Or, "Perhaps this is a necessary, transitory step toward a new type of world civilization." In any case, my argument was not accepted.

Four years ago, I and a group of associates met with Presidential advisors at the White House to discuss U.S. food policies. During our presentation, I said, "Unless we drastically change our direction, within twenty years, this country is going to collapse." I expected them to disagree or to have a different opinion. However, to my surprise, all five advisors nodded in agreement.

I was very happy when, in 1977, the Senate Nutrition Committee released *Dietary Goals for the United States*. This landmark document included the opinions of many conscientious scientists like Dr. Mark Hegsted and Dr. Phillip Lee. Also, I am very happy that macrobiotic people have, for the past fifteen years, taken the initiative in developing the natural foods movement: promoting the use of organic grains, beans, and vegetables, and products such as *tofu, tempeh, natto*, and sea vegetables. Now, nearly 10,000 food stores throughout North America are carrying high quality natural foods. I am also encouraged when many doctors, medical scientists, and researchers publicly advocate dietary change as a means of preventing illness. I can see that after many years of dark struggle, this country is now turning its course and as a result, changing the destiny of modern civilization.

In reality, everyone is their own master. Sickness cannot be blamed on society, on fate, or on heredity. Sickness is caused by what we have been eating and what our ancestors have eaten, and by our day to day thinking and behavior. All of our physical, mental, and social problems stem from these basic causes. If we are sick, the producer of that sickness is no one but us. For example, a condition such as breast cancer is the natural outcome of eating plenty of foods such as ice cream, cheese, and milk; while skin cancer arises from the excessive intake of oily and sugary foods. A person with heart disease should realize that this condition has arisen because he or she has eaten too much meat, too many eggs, and too much sugar. Again, we must ask the question, "Who creates these sicknesses?" The answer is, of course, no one but ourselves. Since we are the creators of our sicknesses, it is up to us to overcome them.

I respect modern medicine very much, but up until now, its primary emphasis has been on the relief of symptoms. If, when someone experiences an abnormal symptom, he goes to the hospital, his doctors will usually try to eliminate it through the injection of drugs or through surgery or other procedures. However, a disease can only be considered "cured" when the person recognizes his part in creating it and decides to change his condition by eliminating the cause of his sickness. In modern terms, we must wait five years to see if a new or similar symptom develops before declaring that a disease has been cured. Even if the symptoms have been temporarily suppressed, however, unless the patient changes his way of eating, behavior, way of thinking, and life-style, a fundamental cure has not taken place.

Recently, a Venezuelan minister of education visited Boston to discuss how macrobiotics could serve in the future of his country. During our conversation I asked what he thought of American food. He immediately replied, "American food is the worst of any that I have eaten throughout the world." I then asked, "Now that the American life-style, including diet, is spreading to your country, what will you do?" He said, "That is why I came to see you. My main concern is to preserve the natural quality of our traditional foods like grains, beans, and vegetables for the health and well-being of our people."

My wife and I recently returned from giving seminars in Spain and Portugal. While in Spain, I saw many sick people who were seeking macrobiotic advice. One Catholic nun, about thirty-five-years old, was among them. She attended my seminars, and when I saw her privately, she confessed that she was suffering from breast cancer. I asked her how many nuns were in her monastery, and she replied that about 300 were living there. I then asked how many had developed cancer and she told me that sixty-nine had developed the disease and out of these, thirty had died. Thirteen women had entered the monastery when she did, and out of this original group, twelve had died from cancer and she was the only one left.

In Lisbon, there are many macrobiotic restaurants. Each one serves about 400 people every day, including many local office workers and company employees. There is also a prison in Portugal where macrobiotic meals are now being served. Out of the 400 prisoners who are there, twenty-two have begun to cook and eat macrobiotically. During the six months that this program has been in effect, a noticeable difference has developed between the twenty-two macrobiotic prisoners and the other inmates. The macrobiotic prisoners now spend time every day studying macrobiotic philosophy and problems of individual and social health. A number of them had committed bank robberies, theft, and arson, but now they want to serve society and help humanity. Their faces are becoming cleaner and clearer, and they have become much more energetic and at the same time more peaceful. When I visited the prison recently, they all told me that they wanted to dedicate themselves to study, hard work, and helping others. The director of the prison agreed completely with their suggestion that macrobiotic meals be made available to all 400 prisoners.

Meanwhile, all of the macrobiotic prisoners have earned special privileges since starting to eat this way, as a result of noticeable improvements in their conduct. They are even allowed to visit their homes on weekends. In comparing these prisoners to the nuns in the monastery it is apparent that we cannot become healthy or happy unless we eat properly, regardless of whether we seem to be good persons or not.

Of course, we have no objection if you decide to eat a gallon of ice cream every night, provided you first register your will at City Hall. Also, we do not mind if you enjoy quarts of sugared soft drinks every day, as long as you have made an appointment with your dentist. But if you want to lower your cholesterol, enjoy more flexibility in mind and body, and experience an improved level of well-being for yourself and your family, please eat properly.

When evaluating your daily diet, please consider the following points:

1. Do I eat unrefined, whole cereal grains every day, and thoroughly chew each mouthful of food?
2. Are my daily foods natural in their quality, and do I avoid heavily processed, highly artificial foods?
3. Do I use fresh vegetables every day?
4. Do I season my daily meals with a moderate amount of mineral-rich sea salt rather than refined table salt?
5. Do I try not to overconsume meat, eggs, cheese, poultry, and other items containing plenty of saturated fat and cholesterol?
6. Do I use high quality, natural grain sweeteners rather than highly refined sugar or concentrated sweeteners like honey and maple syrup?
7. Do I avoid overconsuming fruit or fruit juices, especially those originating in the tropics.

If your answers to these questions include many "no's," may we suggest that you consider the macrobiotic dietary and way of life approach presented in this book.

At present, the recovery of proper food is the most urgent issue in America and the modern world. Beginning with our next meal, let us change toward a more healthy and sound way of eating. Let us also use our daily food to recover the balance of mind, body, and spirit so that our families, our society, and the world may develop in a more peaceful and harmonious direction.

Cancer and Modern Civilization

I recently spoke with a middle aged woman who was suffering from breast cancer. Before learning about our dietary approach, she had already undergone an operation and received about ten radiation treatments. She had taken medication consisting of hormone and vitamin therapy and chemotherapy was now being considered as well. After all of this, she was still considered a borderline case— the cancer had definitely not been controlled.

This woman's case is not unique. Modern medical science has yet to reach any definite conclusions regarding either the cause or treatment of cancer. In fact, there are more cases of cancer now than when concentrated research began over thirty years ago.

During 1980 over 750,000 Americans developed cancer, with 2,100 new cases each day. Over 400,000 cancer patients, 1,100 a day, died. The triumph of modern medicine, which began its development about one hundred years ago, is now reflected in magnificent hospitals, elaborate technologies, and highly trained specialists. But the strength and splendor of all these accomplishments is now being seriously challenged by the problem of cancer.

In the field of cancer research, scientists have pioneered such techniques as surgery, radiation therapy, laser therapy, chemotherapy, hormone therapy, and others—but these treatments are, at best, successful only in achieving temporary relief of symptoms. In the majority of cases, they fail to prevent the disease from recurring, as they do not address the root cause of origin of the problem.

It is already widely known that the rates of cancer, heart disease, diabetes, mental illness and other degenerative diseases have been steadily increasing throughout the century, and in nearly all of the world's populations. In fact, it is becoming apparent that if this rapid expansion of biological decline continues, the civilized world may soon be threatened with widespread collapse.

We believe this collapse is not inevitable; but to prevent such a catastrophe from occurring, we must begin to approach such problems as cancer with a new orientation. We must begin to seek out the most basic causes and to implement the most basic solutions, rather than continue the present approach of treating each problem separately in terms of its symptoms alone.

The problem of degenerative disease affects us all in one way or another. Therefore, the responsibility of finding and implementing solutions should not be left only to those within the medical and scientific communities. It is our belief that the recovery of global health will emerge only through a cooperative effort involving people at all levels of society.

When I came to America more than thirty years ago, cancer was a much more remote problem than it is today. In late 1981, the National Cancer Institute announced that one out of every three Americans will eventually develop the disease during their lifetime. If cancer continues to increase at the present rate,

50 percent of the population will develop the disease by the end of the century; and during the next century, virtually everyone will develop cancer. Rather than being a century of health, peace, and progress, the twenty-first century promises to be the "century of cancer."

A similar situation exists with other chronic and degenerative disorders. Thirty years ago the rate of mental illness in America was one out of twenty; it has now more than doubled to over one out of ten. Obesity is a recognized risk factor in many of our leading causes of death including cardiovascular disease, liver disease, and diabetes; and obesity, like mental illness, can be severely debilitating even when not fatal. One out of every three Americans is now considered to be overweight to a degree that has significantly reduced their life expectancy.

During the Kennedy administration, millions of dollars were allocated for research on the common cold, yet now almost twenty years later, there are still no conclusive results. In fact, no major sicknesses can really be cured by modern methods. In some cases they may be symptomatically controlled, but fundamentally they cannot be cured.

Given these and many other trends, we can clearly see that America, together with our modern civilization as a whole, is now on the verge of self-extinction as a result of deep-seated chronic biological degeneration. The time left to us to reverse this direction is very short. By the time the present generation grows to adulthood, we may be witnessing the complete decline of our recently developed modern way of life; the final collapse may come within the next twenty, or at the most, forty years.

This sad failure, however, can also be seen as an opportunity for deep self-reflection. The cancer problem offers the chance to seriously rethink our present understanding of health and sickness and to examine the basic premises of our way of life.

The modern way of thought, for example, usually regards cancer as an aberration caused by certain factors (e.g., virus, genes, or carcinogenic substances) that are viewed as "enemies." To cure the cancer, these "enemies" must be removed—sought out and destroyed, bombarded by chemicals and radiation. Our modern understanding of life, health, sickness, and the nature of man is *dualistic*. Dualistic thinking divides good from bad, friend from enemy, seeing the one as desirable and the other as undesirable. This divisive mode of thought actually underlies all of modern society, including education and religion, politics and economics, science and industry, and it has culminated in the dead end reached by our modern failure to solve the problem of cancer.

As long as our basic point of view is dualistic, it is impossible to fundamentally cure any sickness, whether diabetes, emphysema, leprosy, arthritis, mental illness, or even the common cold. The current mode of attack stems from our ignorance of the true nature of life and health. In a profound sense, while the riddle of cancer is testing our modern medical understanding, it is also challenging modern civilization itself.

Modern Theories

There are presently two principal theories regarding the cause of cancer. The first is that cancer arises as a result of "cancer-inducing substances" including chemicals and preservatives in food, chemicals and pollutants in the environment such as asbestos or industrial wastes, and external stimuli such as x-rays or ultraviolet rays. The second major explanation is the "virus theory," arrived at through microscopic examination of cancer cells, revealing the presence of virus. The presence of virus cells led to the conclusion that these cells were the cause of the condition, and that cancer might therefore be infectious.

Other factors are also suspect; for instance, some scientists have begun to think that some defect in the genes passed on to an individual at birth can create a predisposition to cancer later in life or, in other words, that the tendency to develop cancer may be hereditary.

However, none of these theories has resulted in the discovery of a comprehensively effective treatment. The principal discovery to date has been that early detection is the most advisable means of controlling the disease. Furthermore, some of the current diagnostic methods may be contributing to accelerated malignant growth. X-ray scanning for breast or lung tumors, for example, is now commonly suspected of increasing the risk of developing a malignancy in the breast.

Once a cancer is detected, *surgical removal* of the cancerous tissue or of an entire diseased organ or gland remains the primary method of treatment. Other widely used treatments include *radiation therapy* (radioactive bombardment of the cancer cells) and *chemotherapy* (the injection of powerful chemicals into the bloodstream). There are also various additional forms of treatment, currently in the experimental stage, such as *thermotherapy* or *hypothermia* (inducing high fever by subjecting the entire body to intensive heat), *immunotherapy* (attempting to stimulate the body's native internal defense mechanisms, usually by injections of vitamin A, Interferon, or other substances), *photoradiation* (the injection and laser-excitation of photo-active materials which may transmute into lethal gases, killing the cancerous cells), or *Laetrile*, the controversial vitamin B_{17}, which has recently been legally adopted for experimentation in the United States.

How effective are these treatments? It is difficult to say with certainty, but the evidence so far is not encouraging. For example, authorities have found that childhood cancer victims, treated with radiation and chemotherapy, stand a greater chance than normal children of developing a new cancer in later years. In general, it is estimated that untreated cancer patients may actually live longer than those who receive treatment.

The Origin of Cancer

The problems of cancer and other degenerative diseases cannot be separated from the problems of modern civilization as a whole. For example, I recently sat on the bench of a Boston Probate Court. It seemed that every five minutes a different couple would enter and receive the judge's consent for a divorce. This continued throughout the day, reminding me of an automobile assembly line.

I met with several of the judges afterward and asked them why the divorce rate was increasing so rapidly. One judge answered, "Traditional values are no longer being taught in schools, nor are they being practiced or respected at home."

Everyone agreed that something should be done to prevent these breakdowns in family relations. One judge mentioned that in the past it was easier to guide couples in the direction of reconciliation; but lately, he went on to say, preventing a divorce had become almost impossible in most cases. Their own efforts, he said, were now directed more toward protecting the welfare of the children. They had also observed that the influence of church or school education, legal restriction or government intervention, no longer seemed capable of reversing this trend. One judge finally concluded that divorce was actually a symptom of our modern civilization itself.

The same can be said of cancer, heart disease, mental illness, and all the degenerative sicknesses. The epidemic of degenerative disease, the decline of traditional human values, and the decomposition of society itself are all indications that something is deeply wrong with modern life. Let us consider the following trends which have helped to create our modern situation.

1. A Materialistic Viewpoint

At present, we tend to view the development of civilization in terms of our advancing material prosperity; at the same time, we tend to undervalue the development of human consciousness and spirit. But this viewpoint is out of proportion with the very nature of existence. The world of matter itself is tiny, almost insignificant, when compared to the vast currents of moving space and energy which envelop it, and out of which it has come into being.

Not only is the material world infinitesimally small by comparison, but also, as modern atomic physics has discovered, the more we analyze it and take it apart, the more we discover that it actually has no concrete existence. In other words, the search for an ultimate unit of matter, which began with Democritus' statement that reality could be divided into "atoms and space," has ended in the twentieth century with the discovery that sub-atomic particles are nothing but highly charged matrixes of moving energy.

However, our senses, which are limited, easily delude us into believing that things have fixed or unchanging quality. For example, all of the cells, tissues, skin, and organs which comprise the human body are continuously changing.[1] As a result, what we think of as today's "self" is very different from yesterday's "self" and tomorrow's "self." This is obvious to parents who have watched their children grow. However, our development does not stop when we reach physical maturity: our consciousness and judgment also change and develop throughout life.

---

[1] It has been calculated that red cells in the bloodstream live about 120 days. In order to maintain a relatively constant number of these cells, an astounding 200,000,000 new cells are cerated every minute, while an equal number of old cells are continuously destroyed.

In reality, there is nothing static, fixed, or permanent; yet modern people frequently adopt an unchanging and inflexible attitude and as a result experience repeated frustration and disappointment when faced with the ephemerality of life. We have all heard stories about people who spent their lives gaining a fortune, only to fall into despair upon discovering that their basic needs are unfulfilled.

2. Commercialism, Artificiality, and a Decline in Quality

Today, the successful production of consumer goods is based largely on marketing them on a mass scale. In order to succeed, a product must in some way stimulate or gratify the senses. Of itself, sensory satisfaction is not necessarily destructive. Everyone is entitled to satisfy his basic needs. However, trouble arises when sensory gratification becomes a society's driving motive. This causes it to degenerate, since the realm of the senses is so limited in comparison to our native capacities of imagination, understanding, compassion, insight, and love.

The quality of food is a good example. In the past, most people appreciated the simple, natural taste and texture of brown bread, brown rice, and other whole natural foods. Now, in order to stimulate the senses, brown rice is usually refined and polished into nutritionally deficient white rice, while whole wheat bread has been replaced by marshmallow-soft white bread.

At the same time, a huge industry has developed to enhance sensory appeal by adding artificial colorings, flavorings, and texture agents to our daily foods. Over the last forty years, this trend has extended to many items necessary for daily living, including clothing, housing materials, furniture, sleeping materials, and kitchen utensils. As many have discovered, however, the application of artificial technology to the production of consumer goods often results in a degradation in quality.

All in all, we are moving toward a totally artificial way of life and have gotten further and further away from our origins in the natural world. However, human life would not exist without the solar system or the earth, or without air, water, or vegetation. By orienting our way of life against nature, we are in effect trying to oppose and ultimately destroy ourselves.

Cancer is only one result of this total orientation. However, instead of considering the larger environmental, societal, and dietary causes of cancer, most research is presently moving in the opposite direction, viewing the disease mainly as an isolated cellular disorder, and most therapies focus only on removing or destroying the cancerous tumor while ignoring the overall bodily condition which caused it to develop.

Cancer generally begins as a growth in one specific area, serving the purpose of detoxifying other bodily functions and organs by localizing the body's overall toxic condition. Therefore, while the cancer is developing, the functioning of the other organs and of the body as a whole is able to continue as normal. Cancer is not a disease, then, of certain cells of certain organs. It is a means of self-protection for an entire diseased organism. By removing this cancerous growth, we then allow the toxins to scatter again throughout the body, creating the conditions for another form of sickness or perhaps another localization.

From a holistic perspective, in other words, cancer is seen as an attempt on the part of the body to establish balance. If the cancer is removed, this balance is disrupted and may collapse.

Of primary importance in dealing with cancer is not to disturb this natural mechanism by taking out or destroying the cancer itself. On the contrary, we must totally affirm and approve of the body's natural efforts to maintain a functioning harmony.

Once we cease our efforts to remove the cancer, we are in a position to ask the all-important question, "What has created this toxic condition?" In considering the question, we cannot ignore the pivotal role of our daily food in determining our physiological condition. Over the past fifty years, as noted above, the types of foods we consume have changed drastically, in composition, quality, processing, and proportion. With the rise of affluence, rich foods such as fatty meats, dairy products, and sugar have become widely available in quantity. Simple, unrefined foods have been overwhelmingly replaced by such items as white bread, orange juice, French fries, cola, processed cheeses and meat products, and a wide range of chemical additives, drugs, and medications.

It is noteworthy that as these foods have become more widely used, the incidences of many types of cancer have risen at a rapid rate. Any and all of these foods may create a chronically toxic blood condition and therefore be responsible for creating cancer. By positively influencing the physiological quality of our blood, cells, lymph, and other body fluids through proper nutrition, we can reverse that toxic quality, and the localization represented by the cancer condition becomes unnecessary. Practically speaking, *potential cancers may be avoided, and existing cancers reversed*, with the correct change in daily food.

More specifically, if we study traditional eating patterns over the past millenium, we find that the human diet has generally consisted of whole cereal grains, beans, and fresh vegetables, supplemented with seasonal fruits, nuts and seeds, small quantities of lean animal foods, and in some areas edible seaweeds and fermented soybean products. Combined with the proper techniques of selection, combination and cooking, these foods do not produce the chronic toxic condition underlying cancer.

Cancer originates long before the formation of a malignant growth and is rooted in the quality of the external factors which we are selecting and consuming. When cancer is finally discovered, however, this external origin is often overlooked, and the disease is considered to be cured as long as the tumor or tumors have been removed or destroyed. However, since the cause has not been changed, the cancer will often return, in either the same or some other location. This is usually met by another round of treatment which again ignores the cause. This type of approach represents an often futile attempt to control only the symptoms of the disease.

In order to control cancer, we need to see beyond the immediate symptom and consider larger factors such as the patient's overall blood quality, the types of foods which have been used to create that blood quality, and the mentality and way of life which have led the patient to select those particular foods. It is also important to see beyond the individual patient and into the realm of society at large. Factors such as the orientation of the food industry, the quality of modern agriculture, and our increasingly unnatural and sedentary way of life play a large part in the problem of cancer.

A Macrobiotic Approach to Cancer

Cancer is not the result of some outside factor over which we have no control. Rather, it is simply the product of our own daily behavior, including our thinking, life-style and way of eating. Why is it, for example, that in considering two people, both living in the same general environment, we find that one develops cancer while the other does not? This must be the result of each person's own unique way of behavior, including all of the above factors.

When we bring these simple considerations into a less extreme, more manageable balance the symptom of cancer is no longer being created. To aid in restoring this balance to our lives, the following practices are beneficial.

1. Self Reflection
Sickness is an indication that our way of life is not harmonious with the environment. To establish genuine health, we must rethink our basic outlook on life. In one sense, sickness results from our arrogance in thinking that life's main purpose is to give us sensory satisfaction, emotional comfort, or material prosperity. As a result of this more limited view, we often place our happiness above that of everyone else, and our daily life frequently becomes more competitive, suspicious, and defensive.

A more natural, harmonious balance can only be established by abandoning egocentric thinking and adopting a more universal attitude. As a first step, we can begin by caring for and offering our love to our parents, family members, friends, and to all people in our society; even extending our love and sympathy to those we think of as our "enemies." This attitude is fundamental to the macrobiotic approach to health.[2]

2. Respect for the Natural Environment
The relationship of man and nature is like that of the embryo and the placenta. The placenta nourishes, supports and sustains the developing embryo. It would be quite bizarre if the embryo were to seek to destroy this protector organism. Likewise, it is simply a matter of common sense that we should strive to preserve the integrity of the natural environment upon which we depend for life itself.

---

[2] In a recent nine-year survey of 7,000 randomly selected adults conducted by researchers at the Yale University School of Medicine, persons with a wide range of social contacts were found to have a better chance of leading a longer life than those with a more limited range of contacts. A solid network of friends, acquaintances, and relatives was found to decrease the probability of dying by a factor of 2.3 among men and 2.8 among the women. (From *Science News*, Vol. 118, January 17, 1981.)

Over the last century, however, we have steadily aggravated the contamination of our soil, water and air. Is this not a self-destructive course?

Our daily way of life has also become more unnatural. Most modern people, for example, watch plenty of television, and especially color television, exposing themselves continually to great quantities of unnatural radiation. Many homes and institutional facilities also now use microwave cooking devices or electric ranges, which actually weaken our natural ability to resist disease.

Most people wear clothes made of synthetic fabrics, such as nylon stockings and undergarments, or polyester shirts. Many people also use sheets, blankets, carpets, and other household items made of synthetic materials. Synthetically produced items such as these interfere with the smooth exchange of energy between our bodies and the environment; naturally, they also contribute to the eventual development of sickness or make the recovery from sickness more difficult.

3. Naturally Balanced Diet

The trillions of cells which comprise the human body are created and nourished by the bloodstream. New blood cells are constantly being manufactured from the nutrients provided by our daily foods. If we eat improperly, the quality of our blood, and therefore of our cells, begins to deteriorate. Cancer, a cellular disorder, is largely the result of improper eating over a long period.

For restoring sound, healthy blood and cell quality, we recommend the following dietary principles:

(1) Harmony with the evolutionary order

When we examine characteristics such as the structure and function of human teeth or the length of the intestine and digestive tract, it is apparent that whole cereal grains comprise the most appropriate principal food for man, followed by local vegetables, beans, and other regional supplements.[3]

(2) Harmony with universal dietary tradition

The modern diet has developed largely over the last fifty years and includes many items which were unknown in the past such as rich, fatty foods, refined sugar, and highly processed or artificial foods. At the same time, mankind's traditional staples—whole cereal grains, beans, and vegetables—are no longer consumed as principal foods. The rising incidence of degenerative disease closely parallels these changes in the human diet.

(3) Harmony with the ecological order

It is advisable to base our diet mostly on foods produced in the same general area in which we live. A traditional people like the Eskimo base their diet mostly on animal products and this is appropriate in a cold polar climate. In India and other more tropical regions, a diet based almost entirely on vegetable-quality foods is more conducive to health. When we begin to eat foods which have been im-

---

[3] For a more thorough discussion of the relation of food to the process of biological evolution, please refer to *The Book of Macrobiotics: The Universal Way of Health and Happiness* by the author, published by Japan Publications, Inc., 1977.

ported from regions with different climatic conditions, a condition of chronic imbalance results, especially when we eat large quantities of sugar, pineapples, bananas, citrus, and other tropical products while living in a temperate climate. Whole cereal grains, beans, local vegetables, and other regional supplements are the ideal principal foods in a temperate climate region.

(4) Harmony with the changing seasons

A habit like eating ice cream in a heated apartment while snow is falling outside is obviously disharmonious with the seasonal order as is consuming charcoal-broiled steaks in the heat of the summer. It is better to naturally adjust the selection and preparation of daily foods to harmonize with the changing seasons. For example, in colder weather we can apply longer cooking times, while minimizing the intake of raw salad or fruit. In the summer, lightly cooked dishes are more appropriate while the intake of animal food and heavily cooked items can be minimized.

(5) Harmony with individual differences

Individual differences need to be considered in the selection and preparation of our daily foods, with variations according to age, sex, type of activity, occupation, original constitution and present condition. We also recommend the following daily considerations:[4]

1. Water—It is preferable to use high quality, clean natural water for cooking and drinking. Spring or well water is fine for regular use; it is best to avoid chemically treated or distilled water.

2. Carbohydrates—It is advisable to eat carbohydrates mostly in the form of polysaccharide glucose, such as that found in cereal grains, vegetables, and beans, while minimizing or avoiding the intake of mono- or disaccharide sugars, such as those in fruit, honey, refined sugar, and other sweeteners.

3. Protein—It is recommended that protein be taken primarily from vegetable sources like whole grains and bean products, while reducing the use of animal proteins.

4. Fat—It is better to avoid the hard, saturated fats found in most types of animal foods. High quality, unsaturated fats such as those in vegetable oils are more appropriate for regular use.

5. Salt—It is better to rely primarily on natural sea salt, which contains a variety of trace minerals, and to avoid refined salt, which is almost 100 percent sodium chloride with no trace minerals.

In a temperate, four-season climate, an optimum daily diet consists of about 50 to 60 percent whole cereal grains, 5 percent soup (one or two small bowls), preferably seasoned with *miso* or *tamari* soy sauce; 25 to 30 percent vegetables prepared in a variety of styles; and 5 to 10 percent beans and sea vegetables. Supplementary foods include occasional locally grown fruits, preferably cooked;

---

[4] These recommendations closely parallel those made over the last five years by the Nutrition Subcommittee of the U.S. Senate, the Surgeon General of the United States, the U.S. Department of Health and Welfare, the National Academy of Sciences, and many leading international health agencies.

seafood; and a variety of seeds and nuts. (A more detailed description of the Standard Macrobiotic Diet is presented later in this chapter.)

4. *An Active Daily Life*
For many of us, modern life offers fewer physically and mentally challenging circumstances than in the past. As a result, functions such as the circulation of blood and lymph, and the activity of the digestive and nervous systems often stagnate. However, a physically and mentally active life is essential for good health. Therefore, it is advisable to supplement the more regulated patterns of modern life with regular physical and mental exercise.

Medically Terminal or Macrobiotically Hopeful?

I have met thousands of cancer patients over the last fifteen years. Of these, 90 percent or more had already received chemotherapy, radiation, or some other treatment. Many were considered terminal. In some cases there was nothing that medicine could do for them; in others, all possible treatments had already been tried, with no success.

Patients who have received treatment often take longer to recover than those who have not, and their recovery is often more complicated and difficult. With macrobiotics, we try to change the quality of the blood and cells through the most natural methods. However, when violent or artificial treaments have first been applied, a person must recover not only from the cancer but also from the toxic and unnatural effects of the treatment.

This brings us to the difference between cases which are considered to be *medically terminal* and those which are considered *macrobiotically terminal*. A medically terminal case is one for which present treatments offer no hope of recovery. In some cases, an exploratory operation is performed and the patient is told that no treatment will be applied. Persons in this situation often have a better possibility of recovery than those who are considered hopeful and who receive radiation, chemotherapy, surgery, or some other form of treatment. A number of factors which also interfere with the natural process of recovery are summarized below:

1. *Lack of Gratitude*
Persons who are ungrateful frequently say things like, "Why should I eat this brown rice? Why do I have to eat these tasteless vegetables?" or "How long do I have to stay on this diet?" An ungrateful person never thinks that he himself might have created his cancer but usually believes instead that it is the unfair result of some unknown external factor. When someone with this attitude begins macrobiotics, they frequently return to their previous diet of meat, sugar, eggs, cheese, and other similar foods as soon as some improvement is experienced.

2. *Inaccurate Dietary Practice*
In some cases, the macrobiotic dietary recommendations are not well understood

or carefully practiced. For example, when recommendations such as "eat 50 to 60 percent whole grains every day, prepare rice in a pressure cooker and add a pinch of sea salt to it," are presented, most people indicate that they understand. However, upon returning home, some might cook with too much salt or with no salt, or with too much water or not enough; or they may boil or bake rather than pressure-cook. Some people might even eat 100 percent grain instead of 50 to 60 percent. Naturally, this type of practice hinders their recovery.

When we advise further study of macrobiotic cooking, some people reply that they already know how to cook. However, their previous style of cooking was one of the major factors which caused their cancer to develop. Persons who feel they already know how to cook often have more difficulty with macrobiotics since they must forget their previous knowledge and start from the beginning.

3. Lack of Will
In some cases, persons who have no desire to live are introduced to macrobiotics, often by some other well-intentioned person. Persons such as this, who frequently ignore the advice they are given, have a very slight chance of recovering.

4. Lack of Family Support
Among the many patients that I have counseled were many middle-aged gentlemen who, although they were married, visited by themselves. When asked why their wives had not come, they often replied that their wives did not agree with their wish to begin macrobiotics. When asked who would cook, more often than not they replied that they would try to do it. I have also met many women who did not have the support of their husbands.

I sympathize very much with people like this because, in the real sense, they are alone. Their families lack the love and care that are essential for their recovery.

Of all the patients I have met, those who recovered were either single or had the full support of their families, even to the extent that the other family members also started macrobiotics and learned how to cook and care for the patient. Therefore, if you wish to begin macrobiotics and your husband or wife is against the idea, you might investigate the possibility of a temporary separation, at least until you recover. Someone who refuses to help their partner regain life, health, and happiness is no longer a true spouse.

5. Loss of Natural Healing Ability
Extensive chemotherapy or radiation tend to diminish the body's self-healing abilities and interfere with the natural process of recovery. If a person has completely lost their self-healing abilities through such treatments, it is doubtful that macrobiotics can help them recover.

A case can be considered macrobiotically terminal when any of these factors are present regardless of the actual stage of the tumor. However, it is still worthwhile for persons such as these to begin macrobiotics, since it can help reduce much unnecessary pain and suffering. There have been several instances in which people who had terminal conditions started macrobiotics. After several weeks they became very peaceful and experienced the disappearance of pain. Then, when the end came, they were able to die in a more peaceful and dignified manner.

When a person first hears about macrobiotics, he or she might lack confidence in it because it seems new. If, as a result the person decides to pursue macrobiotics along with conventional therapy, recovery might be slower. This combined appraoch can work temporarily, but once a patient starts to improve it is better to begin reducing the frequency of outside treatment over a period of from one to four months.

If surgery is considered during this time, it is better to limit it to that which is absolutely necessary—for example, situations such as those in which a tumor completely blocks the passage of food through the digestive tract. Since partial blockages of the digestive system can be remedied through macrobiotics, surgery is advisable only in emergency situations.

Diet and the Development of Cancer

When cancer develops, a greenish shade will often appear on the skin. The appearance of this color represents a process of biological degeneration. To better understand this, let us consider the order of colors in the biological world.

Among the seven primary colors, red has the longest wave length and is more yang. The opposite colors—purple, blue, and green—have shorter wave lengths and are cooler. We therefore classify them as more yin.[5] Red is the color of the more yang animal kingdom and is readily apparent in the color of the blood. On

Fig. 1 **The Relationship between Color and the Development of Cancer: The Biological Processes of Humanization (I) and Cell Decomposition (II)**

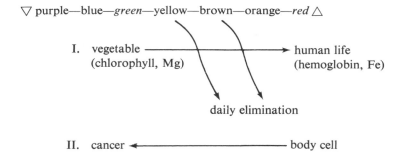

The above diagram depicts the classification of basic colors from yin ($\triangledown$) to yang ($\triangle$). The process of humanization (I) represents the transformation of green vegetable life into human blood and body cells. Cancer represents a reverse process (II) in which body cells decompose, often producing a greenish shade on the skin.

---

[5] For an explanation of the principles of yin and yang, please refer to *The Book of Macrobiotics: The Universal Way of Health and Happiness* by the author, published by Japan Publications, Inc., 1977.

Fig. 2 Correlations between Greenish Discolorations and Cancer Types

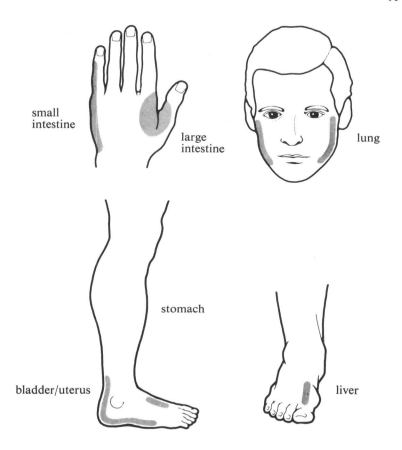

the other hand, more yin vegetables are based on green chlorophyll. Eating represents the process whereby we transform green vegetable life into red animal blood. It is based on the ability to change magnesium, which lies at the center of the chlorophyll molecule, into iron, the element which forms the basis of hemoglobin.

The more yin colors—purple and blue—appear in the sky and atmosphere, both of which are more expanded or yin components of the environment. The more yang colors—yellow, brown, and orange—appear in the more compacted world of minerals. During the transformation of vegetable life into human blood and cells, waste products are eliminated through functions such as urination and bowel movements. These represent in between stages in the transformation of vegetable into human life and therefore are yellow and brown, colors which lie in between green and red in the spectrum. Cancer represents a reverse process in which body cells decompose and change back toward vegetable life, and is manifested in the greenish shade appearing on the skin.

In the case of colon cancer, for example, this color might appear on the outside of either hand in the indented area between the thumb and forefinger (see Fig. 2).

Several other examples are listed below.[6]

Cancer Type	Region Where Greenish Shade Might Appear
Small Intestine	Outside of the little finger
Lung	Either or both cheeks
Stomach	Along the outside front of either leg, especially below the knee
Bladder/Uterine	Around either ankle on the outside of the leg
Liver	Around the top of the foot in the central area

To further understand how cancer develops, we can use the analogy of a tree (see Fig. 3). A tree has a structure which is opposite to the human body. For example, body cells have a more closed structure and are nourished by red blood, while the leaves of a tree, which correspond to the body's cells, have a more expanded structure and a green color. A tree's life-blood comes from the nutrients absorbed through external roots. The roots of the body lie deep in the intestines

Fig. 3   Comparison between a Tree and the Human Body

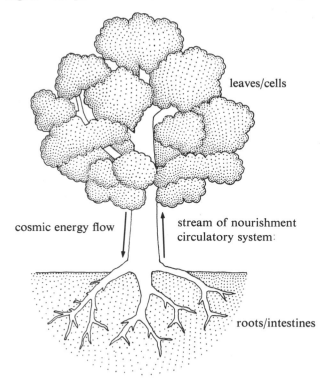

leaves/cells

cosmic energy flow

stream of nourishment
circulatory system:

roots/intestines

---

[6] For additional correlations, please refer to *Natural Healing through Macrobiotics* (*1979*) and *How to See Your Health: The Book of Oriental Diagnosis* (*1980*) by the author, published by Japan Publications, Inc.

in the region where nutrients are absorbed into the blood and then distributed to all of the body's cells. If the quality of nourishment is chronically poor, however, cells eventually lose their normal functioning ability as the quality of the cellular environment begins to deteriorate. This condition results from the repeated intake of poor nutrients and does not arise suddenly. While it is developing, many other symptoms might arise in other parts of the body. Therefore, cancer develops over time out of a chronically pre-cancerous state. In my estimation, as many as 80 to 90 percent of the American people have some type of pre-cancerous condition.

The repeated overconsumption of certain foods causes the body to make a variety of adjustments in normal functions like elimination and respiration. It undergoes chronic discharges and begins the pre-cancerous storage of excess. Several of these processes are outlined below:

1. Normal Discharge
If we eat a reasonable volume of high quality food and maintain an active daily life, normal biological functions—urination, bowel movements, respiration, perspiration, etc.—efficiently discharge any excess. Discharge also takes place through daily thinking and activity, as well as through normal functions like menstruation, childbirth and lactation.

2. Abnormal Discharge
However, practically everyone eats and drinks excessively, and this often triggers a variety of abnormal discharge mechanisms such as diarrhea, overly frequent bowel movements, or frequent urination beyond the normal three to four times per day. Habits like scratching the head, tapping the feet, and frequent blinking also represent abnormal discharges, as do emotions such as anger. Periodically, excess is discharged through more acute symptoms such as a sudden fever, coughing, or sneezing.

3. Chronic Discharge
Chronic discharges are the next stage in this process and often take the form of skin diseases. These are common in cases where the kidneys have lost their ability to properly cleanse the bloodstream. For example, skin markings such as freckles and dark spots indicate the chronic discharge of sugar and other simple carbohydrates, while white patches indicate the discharge of milk, cottage cheese, and other dairy products.

Hard, dry skin arises after the bloodstream fills with fat and oil, eventually causing blockage of the pores, hair follicles, and sweat glands. When these blockages prevent the flow of liquid toward the surface, the skin becomes dry. Many people believe that this condition results from a lack of oil, when in fact it is caused by the intake of too much fat and oil.

4. Accumulation
If we continue to eat poorly, we eventually exhaust the body's ability to discharge. This can be serious if an underlying layer of fat has developed under the skin

which prevents discharge toward the surface of the body. This condition is caused by the repeated overconsumption of milk, cheese, eggs, and other fatty, oily, or greasy foods.

When this stage has been reached, internal deposits of mucus or fat begin to form, initially in areas which have some direct access to the outside. These deposits frequently develop in the following regions (see Fig. 4):

Fig. 4   Frequent Sites of Mucus and Fat Accumulation in the Body

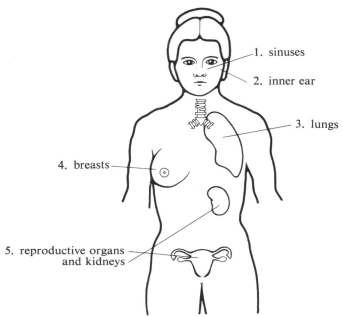

1. sinuses
2. inner ear
3. lungs
4. breasts
5. reproductive organs and kidneys

1. Sinuses—The sinuses are a frequent site of mucus accumulation, and symptoms such as allergies, hay fever, and blocked sinuses often result. Hay fever and sneezing arise when dust or pollen stimulate the discharge of this excess, while calcified stones often form deep within the sinuses. Thick, heavy deposits of mucus in the sinuses diminish our mental clarity and alertness.

2. Inner Ear—The accumulation of mucus and fat in the inner ear interferes with the smooth functioning of the inner ear mechanism and can lead to frequent pain, impaired hearing, and even deafness. About 12 million Americans are now deaf, and this number is steadily increasing, while millions more suffer from impaired hearing.

3. Lungs—Various forms of excess often accumulate in the lungs. Aside from the obvious symptoms of coughing and chest congestion, mucus often fills the alveoli, or air sacs, and breathing becomes more difficult. Occasionally, a coat of mucus in the bronchi can be loosened and discharged by coughing, but once the sacs are surrounded, it becomes more firmly lodged and can remain there for years. Then, if air pollutants or cigarette smoke enter the lungs, their heavier components are attracted to and remain in this sticky environment. In severe cases these deposits can trigger the development of lung cancer. However, the underlying cause of this condition is the accumulation of sticky fat and mucus in the alveoli and in the blood and capillaries which surround them.

4. *Breasts*—The accumulation of excess in this region often results in a hardening of the breasts and the formation of cysts. Excess usually accumulates here in the form of mucus and deposits of fatty acid, both of which take the form of a sticky or heavy liquid. These deposits develop into cysts in the same way that water solidifies into ice, and this process is accelerated by the intake of ice cream, cold milk, soft drinks, orange juice, and similar foods which produce a cooling or freezing effect.

Women who breastfeed their babies are less likely to develop breast cysts or cancer. Women who do not nurse miss this opportunity to discharge through the breasts and therefore face a greater possibility of excess accumulating in this region.

5. *Reproductive Organs and Kidneys*—The prostate gland is a frequent site of accumulation. As a result, it often becomes enlarged, and hard fat deposits or cysts form within and around it. This is one of the principal causes of impotence.

Since the female reproductive organs form a channel leading to the outside of the body, they are a more frequent site for the accumulation of excess as the body attempts to discharge it. This excess can lead to the formation of ovarian cysts as well as to the blockage of the Fallopian tubes. In many cases mucus or fat in the ovaries or Fallopian tubes prevents the passage of the egg and sperm, resulting in an inability to conceive as well as chronic vaginal discharge. Problems with the female sexual organs have become so widespread in America that, in a recent survey, 50 percent of all American women were found to have had a hysterectomy by the age of sixty.

Deposits of mucus and fat also accumulate in the kidneys. These deposits clog the fine network of cells in the interior of the kidneys and cause them to hold water and become chronically swollen. Since elimination is hampered, fluid which cannot be discharged is often deposited in the legs, producing periodic swelling and weakness. If someone with this condition consumes a large quantity of foods which have a chilling effect, the deposited fat and liquid will often crystallize into kidney stones.

Although these symptoms seem unrelated, they all stem from the same underlying cause. However, modern medicine often does not have this view. For example, when someone with a hearing problem or cataracts visits a hospital, they are often referred to an ear or eye specialist. In reality, a symptom such as cataracts indicates a variety of related problems, including mucus accumulation in the breasts, kidneys, and sexual organs.

If, beyond this point, a person continues to eat excessively, the deeper internal organs start to be affected. One common example is the accumulation of cholesterol and saturated fat in and around the heart and in the arteries. If a person reaches the stage where all of the major organs contain heavy deposits and discharge through the skin is blocked by a layer of fat, the result is often obesity and toxic, acidic blood.

An organism cannot survive in this condition. In order to prevent immediate collapse, toxins are localized, leading to the formation of a degenerative cell. As long as improper nourishment is taken in, the body will continue localizing toxins, resulting in the continual growth of the cancer. When a particular location can no longer absorb toxic excess, the body must search for another place to localize it, and so the cancer spreads. This continues until the cancer spreads throughout the body and the person eventually dies.

Symptoms like vaginal discharges, ovarian cysts, hardening of the breasts, skin discharges, dry skin, and similar problems all represent pre-cancerous conditions. However, they need not develop into cancer if we change our way of eating.

Diagnosing Pre-Cancerous Conditions

Pre-cancerous conditions can be diagnosed through careful observation of the eye-whites.[7] Pre-cancerous conditions often correlate with the following markings:

Fig. 5 Eye—White Markings

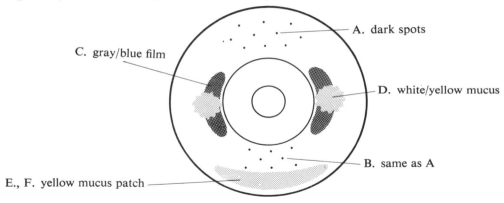

C. gray/blue film

A. dark spots

D. white/yellow mucus

B. same as A

E., F. yellow mucus patch

A. Calcified deposits in the sinuses are frequently indicated by dark spots in the upper portion of the eye-white.

B. Kidney stones and ovarian cysts are often indicated by dark spots in the lower eye-white.

C., D. The accumulation of mucus and fat in the centrally located organs (liver, gallbladder, spleen, and pancreas) frequently appears in the form of a blue, green, or brownish shade, or white patches, in the eye-white on either side of the iris. This often indicates a reduced functioning in these organs.

E. Accumulations of fat and mucus in and around the prostate are often indicated by a yellow coating on the lower part of the eyeball.

F. Fat and mucus accumulations in the female sex organs are frequently indicated

---

[7] For a more thorough explanation of this and other traditional methods of diagnosis, refer to *How to See Your Health: The Book of Oriental Diagnosis* by the author, published by Japan Publications, Inc., 1980.

by a yellow coating in the same area of the eye as E. above. Vaginal discharges, ovarian cysts, fibroid tumors, and similar disorders are also possibly indicated.

Yin and Yang in the Development of Cancer

Yin and yang refer to the two primary forces or tendencies which exist throughout the universe. In the human body, for example, the two branches of the autonomic nervous system—the orthosympathetic and parasympathetic—work in an antagonistic yet complementary manner to control the body's automatic functions. The endocrine system functions in a similar way. The pancreas, for example, secretes insulin, which controls the blood sugar level, and also secretes anti-insulin, which causes it to rise.

Among sicknesses, some are caused by an overly expanding tendency, others from an overly contracting tendency. Still others result from an excessive combination of both. In the Orient, the more expanding tendency is referred to as *yin*, while the opposite, more consolidating tendency is called *yang*.[8]

An example of a more yang sickness is a headache caused when the tissues and cells of the brain contract and press against each other, resulting in pain; while a more yin headache arises when the tissues and cells press against each other as the result of swelling or expansion. Therefore, similar symptoms can arise from opposite causes.

Epilepsy is a more yin disorder caused by the overconsumption of soda, fruit juice, coffee, and other liquids, as well as sugar and other foods which turn into liquid after being eaten. This disorder can be readily controlled by eliminating or minimizing the intake of these items.[9]

Cancer is characterized by a rapid increase in the number of cells, and in this respect, is a more expansive or yin phenomenon. However, the cause of cancer is more complex. As everyone knows, cancer can appear almost anywhere in the body. Skin, brain, liver, uterine, colon, lung, and bone cancer are just a few of the more common types. Each type has a slightly different cause.

To better understand this, let us consider the difference between prostate and breast cancer, both of which are increasing in incidence. Recently, female hormones

---

[8] The terms "yin" and "yang" ("Yō" in Japanese) have been used commonly in the Orient for thousands of years. For example, the terms *Yin-Kyoku* and *Yō-Kyoku* are frequently used in the modern study of electricity and magnetism to describe a negative and a positive charge or magnetic pole. At the same time, an electron is called *Yin-Denshi*, or "yin electric particle," and a proton is called *Yō-Denshi*, or "yang particle." These terms are used frequently in daily conversation.

[9] An example of physiological changes which occur from alterations in yin and yang balance can be seen in the phenomenon known as *hemolysis*. When red blood cells are placed in water (more yin), they swell and finally burst. If they are placed in a 0.9 percent saline solution (more balanced), they remain unchanged, since the concentration of salt in the solution is about the same as the total concentration of salts in the blood plasma and in the red cell itself. If red cells are placed in a more concentrated (yang) solution, for example, 2 percent salt, water begins to leave the cells and they shrink and shrivel.

have been used to temporarily control prostate cancer. At the same time, a male hormone has been found to have a similar controlling effect on breast cancer.

Suppose, however, that female hormones were given to women with breast cancer. This would cause their cancers to develop more rapidly, while male hormones would accelerate the growth of prostate cancer. Therefore, women who have taken birth control pills containing estrogen have a higher risk of developing breast cancer.

As we can see in the above example, breast and prostate cancer have opposite causes. Since more yin female hormones help neutralize prostate cancer, we can assume that this condition is caused by an excess of yang factors. Since breast cancer can be temporarily neutralized by more yang male hormones, this disorder has an opposite, or more yin, cause. Cancers of the stomach, esophagus, and mouth are similar to breast cancer in that their primary cause is an excess of more yin factors, while cancers of the lower digestive tract and prostate are generally caused by excess of more yang factors.

In general, more yin cancers are accelerated by the intake of more yin or expansive foods such as sugar, fruit, dairy products (especially milk and light cheese), oil, flour (especially white flour), alcohol, drugs, coffee, tea, honey, maple sugar and other sweets, chemicals, potatoes, tomatoes, and spices. On the other hand, more yang cancers are accelerated by the repeated overconsumption of more yang or contractive foods including meat, salt, eggs, hard salty cheeses, poultry, and fish.

In an attempt to learn more about the possible causes of different types of cancer, researchers have repeatedly turned to comparative studies of disease rates among different population groups. From our perspective, many of these epidemiological studies reveal interesting relationships between different dietary patterns —the emphasis of certain foods over others—and certain types of cancer.

For example, a 1963 study comparing incidence rates of common cancers among Japanese and American people revealed some startling figures: the Americans were developing over twice as many breast cancers and over three times as many colon cancers as the Japanese—yet the Japanese were suffering with more than six times as many cases of stomach cancer (Table 1).

Another study compared cancer incidence among American White, Black, Chinese and Japanese populations all living in California between 1969 and 1973, with similarly interesting results (Table 2).

These figures clearly reveal different eating habits. Within the general modern dietary pattern of high fats, sugar, refined and artificial foods, there are distinct variations. The Japanese tendency toward stomach cancer is specifically linked to an emphasis on refined cereals such as white rice, together with sugar, vinegar, MSG, and other chemicalized, artificial seasonings.

It is interesting to note the extraordinarily high rate of throat cancers among the Chinese, due largely to their high intake of foods combining oil and fat with sugar, chemicals, and spices, all of which are more yin factors. More cancers in America appear in the lower digestive tract, while those of Orientals are more concentrated in the higher regions.

Table 1 Common Cancers in American and Japanese Populations

Type of cancer	Incidence per 10,000					
	Japanese			American		
	male	female	total	male	female	total
Stomach	49.1	37.6	86.7	7.7	5.6	13.3
Colon	2.1	3.1	6.2	9.3	13.0	22.3
Breast	0.0	4.0	4.0	0.2	9.2	9.4

Table 2 Common Cancers in Various U.S. Population Groups

Type of Cancer	Incidence per 10,000											
	White			Black			Chinese			Japanese		
	M	F	Tot.	M	F	Tot.	M	F	Tot.	M	F	Tot.
Colon	32.7	27.3	60.0	28.1	23.8	51.9	27.5	15.9	43.4	16.0	22.5	38.5
Breast	0.8	88.7	89.5	1.5	64.5	66.0	0.4	49.1	49.5	0.0	44.1	44.1
Ovarian	—	15.1	15.1	—	10.2	10.2	—	7.3	7.3	—	6.0	6.0
Throat	0.8	0.4	1.2	1.2	0.4	1.6	21.8	7.4	29.2	1.0	0.0	1.0

Between 1947 and 1974, milk consumption in Japan jumped twenty-three times; egg consumption increased thirteen times. Meat and other popular American foods have become much more common, and the Japanese diet as a whole has changed rapidly in imitation of the West. As a result, stomach cancer has been reduced by one-third—but colon and breast cancer have risen sharply to approach American rates. A similar situation occurs with Japanese immigrants to America; after three generations of the new environment and new dietary habits, the cancer rates for colon and stomach automatically adjust to conform to the American standards (Fig. 6). This, in fact, was one of the first pieces of epidemiological evidence that the "hereditary theory" might be wrong.

Fig. 6 Mortality Trends: Japanese Migrants to the U.S.
(Haenszel and Kurihara, 1968)

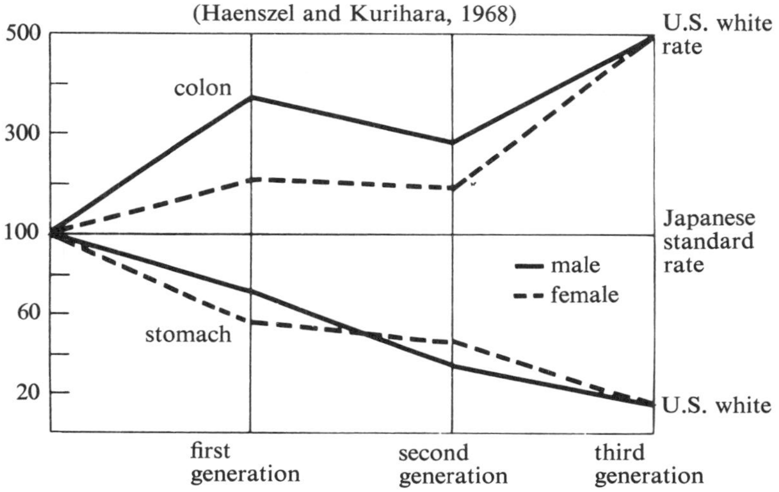

Fig. 7   Opposing Tendencies of Oriental and American Cancers

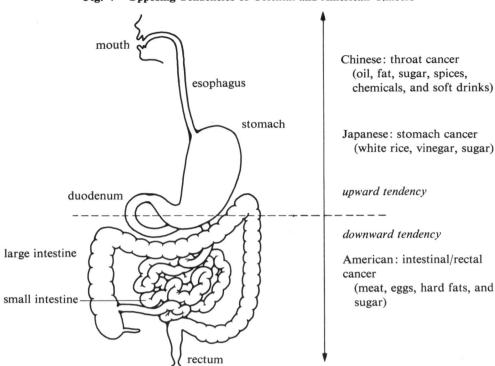

mouth

esophagus

stomach

Chinese: throat cancer
(oil, fat, sugar, spices,
chemicals, and soft drinks)

Japanese: stomach cancer
(white rice, vinegar, sugar)

duodenum

upward tendency

downward tendency

large intestine

American: intestinal/rectal
cancer
(meat, eggs, hard fats, and
sugar)

small intestine

rectum

The Japanese tend to develop more stomach cancers because they eat a large amount of sugar, chemicals, and more yin, chemically grown and treated white rice. Americans develop more colon cancers largely because of a high intake of meat, eggs, and other more yang items. Of course, yin and yang foods are always eaten in combination. But certain people eat a larger volume of one while some eat a larger volume of the other. A woman develops breast cancer largely through the overconsumption of more yin foods, especially milk, sugar, fruit, and fruit juice; while prostate cancer develops largely from the excessive intake of eggs, meat, salty cheese, poultry, and other more yang items.

Fig. 7 illustrates the connection between foods of different populations, and various cancers of the digestive tract.

In general, more yang cancers appear in the lower, deeper parts of the body, usually involving more compacted organs, while more yin cancers usually develop in the higher or more peripheral parts of the body, or in hollow organs. In the case of the large intestine, for example, which is lower and deeper in the body, cancers appearing in the *rectum* and *descending colon*, the more yang parts, are more yang; cancers of a more yin origin arise in the more yin *transverse* and *ascending colons*. Fig. 8 shows the distribution of these four types of large intestinal cancer in Americans.

As another example, the stomach may also be divided into a more yin and a more yang region. While the stomach as a whole is a more yin organ, various types of cancer may develop in different parts of the stomach (Fig. 9).

Fig. 8   Percent Breakdown of U.S. Colon Cancers

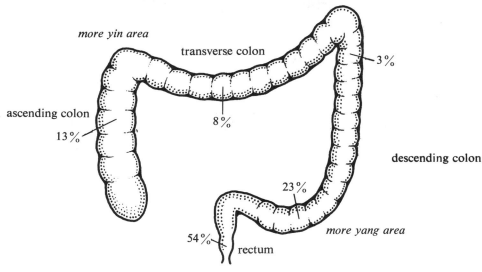

Fig. 9   Complementary Regions of the Stomach

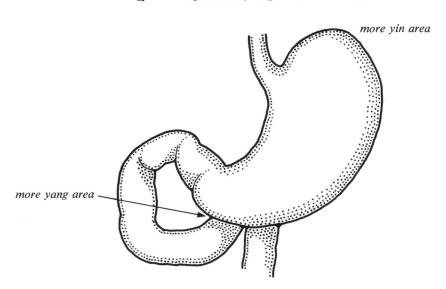

It should be noted that both extreme yin and extreme yang factors are involved in the formation of cancer, although one or the other always predominates. Despite a diet high in meat for instance, the Eskimos rarely developed cancer until refined sugar was introduced into their diet, providing the yin impetus for cancer's rapid growth.

To summarize, some cancers can result from an excess of more extremely yin foods, others from an excess of more extremely yang items, and others from an excess of both extremes. A chart listing common varieties of cancer and their classification according to yin and yang is presented below:

Table 3   General Yin and Yang Classification of Cancer Sites

More yin cause	More yang cause	Yin and yang combined
Breast	Colon	Lung
Stomach	Prostate	Bladder
Skin	Rectum	Uterus
Mouth (except tongue)	Ovary	Kidney
Esophagus	Bone	Spleen
Leukemia	Pancreas	Melanoma
Hodgkin's Disease	Brain (inner regions)	Tongue
Brain (outer regions)		

What are known as carcinogenic factors can also be understood in terms of yin and yang. For example, a number of years ago, tar was suspected as a cancer-causing agent. In order to prove this hypothesis, a group of Japanese scientists repeatedly applied tar to the ears of rabbits. After many days of continued application, cancer started to develop, and it was decided that tar must be a carcinogenic agent. However, tar is not in and of itself a cancer-causing factor. Tar is a more condensed or yang compound. By continuously applying a more yang factor such as this to the rabbit's skin, the cells became inflamed by drawing yin factors from the bloodstream and the inflammation started to spread. This is simply an illustration of the natural law "at the extreme, yang produces yin; while at the extreme, yin will also produce yang."[10]

Similarly, the sun has often been accused of causing skin cancer. However, of itself, the sun is not the cause of this disorder. Repeated exposure to a more yang factor, such as the sun, might trigger a proliferation of cells, especially when foods such as oil, fat, sugar, milk, cola, and other extremely yin items are eaten daily. These foods provide the underlying basis for skin cancer, a more yin disorder, to develop; the yang factor of sunlight serves only as a catalyst to localize these factors on the skin.

Several years ago it was discovered that the fat and protein molecules contained in grilled meat or fish often change into cancerous cells. However, people have eaten foods such as grilled sardines, fish, and meat for thousands of years, yet they rarely developed cancer. Traditionally, these foods were eaten together with plenty of fresh green vegetables, creating a complementary balance which prevented cancer from developing.

---

[10] Other familiar examples are the activation and subsequent expansion (yin) of atoms and molecules following exposure to heat (yang) and the slowing down and subsequent condensation (yang) of atoms and molecules following exposure to cold (yin).

The Standard Macrobiotic Diet

To help offset the development of cancer, it is important to recover a more moderate balance in the daily diet. A more centrally balanced diet based on foods such as whole cereal grains, beans, and cooked vegetables (Fig. 10) can therefore support the recovery from both more yin and more yang cancers.

Fig. 10   The Standard Macrobiotic Diet

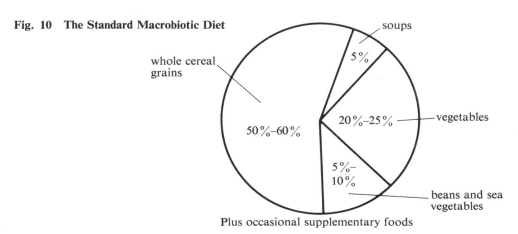

Plus occasional supplementary foods

   This does not mean, however, that the same dietary program should be adopted in every case. Various adjustments are advisable in every circumstance. Before considering these adjustments, however, let us first review the centrally balanced, Standard Macrobiotic Diet. Please keep in mind that these guidelines do not represent medical advice and are not intended to replace personal study with a qualified macrobiotic advisor.

1. Whole Cereal Grains
We recommend that whole cereal grains comprise 50–60 percent of every meal. Whole grains include brown rice, millet, whole wheat, oats, rye, corn, barley, and buckwheat. Please note that whole grains are preferable to flour products, as flour products tend to be more difficult to digest and can be mucus-producing.

2. Soup
One or two cups or small bowls of soup may be included in the daily diet, especially those seasoned with *miso*, *tamari*, or *shoyu*.[11] We recommend that soup

---

[11] *Miso* is processed from soybeans, cereal grains (such as barley, rice or wheat) and sea salt. It is naturally aged and allowed to ferment for more than one-and-a-half years. *Miso* is used in a paste form, and *tamari* soy sauce is used in a liquid form. Both are processed from similar ingredients and have been used for many centuries throughout the Orient. In traditional usage, "*tamari*" means the thick liquid squeezed from fermented *miso*, but in macrobiotics it is used to distinguish traditionally processed, natural soy sauce from commercially available varieties which are artificially processed. Recently, the word "*shoyu*" has been used to denote natural soy sauce as distinguished from *tamari*. *Miso, tamari,* and *shoyu* are available in most natural food stores.

not taste overly salty, and that it contain a variety of suitable vegetables (see below). *Wakame* seaweed can also be included on a daily basis. Soups made with whole grains and beans can also be served from time to time.

3. Vegetable Dishes
Vegetable dishes may comprise 25 to 30 percent of daily intake. Vegetables for daily use include green cabbage, kale, collard and mustard greens, Swiss chard, watercress, bok choy, dandelion, burdock root, carrots, *daikon* radish, turnips and their green tops, onions, acorn, Hubbard, and butternut squash, radish, cauliflower, and others that are locally grown.

It is better to avoid tomatoes, eggplant, potatoes, asparagus, spinach, sweet potatoes, beets, zucchini, yams, avocados, green and red peppers, and other highly acidic varieties.

Vegetables may be prepared in a variety of ways, including boiling, steaming, and sautéeing. Persons with cancer might wish to limit their intake of oil by avoiding deep-fried foods and by restricting their use of oil in sautéeing vegetables to about twice a week.

In general, up to one-third of vegetable intake may be eaten in the form of salad. (It is better to avoid mayonnaise and commercial salad dressings.) However, persons with cancer might need to limit their intake of raw salad. A small amount of salad may be eaten on occasion by those with more yang types of cancer, while it is not advisable for persons with more yin varieties of cancer or cancers caused by an excess of both factors.

4. Beans and Sea Vegetables
About 5 to 10 percent of daily intake may include cooked beans and sea vegetables. However, since beans in general contain much fat and protein, it is advisable for persons with cancer to eat a small quantity of varieties which are lower in fat such as *azuki* beans, chickpeas, and lentils. Naturally processed soybean products such as *tofu*, *tempeh*, and *natto* may be included from time to time depending on the specific condition.

Mineral-rich sea vegetables can be used on a daily basis in soups, with beans, or as side-dishes. Sea vegetables such as *hijiki*, *kombu*, *wakame*, *nori*, dulse, Irish moss, and *alaria* are fine for regular use.

5. Supplementary Foods
Persons in good health may wish to include additional supplementary foods. Among these, a small volume of white meat fish may be eaten once or twice per week. White meat fish generally contains less fat than red meat or blue skin varieties. A small amount of cooked fruit dessert, as well as some fresh and dried fruit, may also be eaten on occasion. It is advisable to eat only locally grown fruits. Thus, if you live in a temperate zone, avoid tropical and semi-tropical fruit (oranges, bananas, pineapples, etc.). It is generally advisable to limit fruit intake to several times a week, while snacks made from roasted seeds, grains, or beans, lightly seasoned with *tamari*, may be enjoyed from time to time.

6. Beverages
Recommended daily beverages include *bancha* (*kukicha*) twig tea, roasted brown rice tea, roasted barley tea, dandelion tea, and cereal grain coffee. Any traditional tea that does not have an aromatic, fragrant, or a stimulant effect can also be used.

7. Additional Suggestions
Cooking oil. If you wish to improve your health, use only high quality sesame or corn oil in moderate amounts.

Salt. Naturally processed, mineral-rich sea salt and traditional, non-chemicalized *miso* and *tamari* soy sauce may be used as seasonings. It is recommended that daily meals not have an overly salty flavor.

The following *condiments* are also recommended for regular use:

(1) *Gomashio* (sesame salt). 10 to 12 parts roasted sesame seeds to 1 part sea salt ground together in a small earthenware bowl called a *suribachi*.

(2) Roasted *kombu* or *wakame* powder. Bake *kombu* or *wakame* in the oven until black. Crush in a *suribachi* and store in a jar or small container.

(3) *Umeboshi* plum[12]

(4) *Tekka*[13]

You may eat regularly two to three times per day, as much as you want, provided that the proportion is correct and chewing is thorough. Please avoid eating for approximately three hours before sleeping. For thirst, use any of the beverages mentioned above or drink small amounts of water (preferably springwater) which is not icy cold.

Adjusting the Standard Diet

When properly applied, the Standard Macrobiotic Diet can help to restore an excessively yin or yang condition to one of more natural balance. However, slight modifications are needed in every case. A few sample modifications for more yin or more yang varieties of cancer are presented in Table 4.

If you are generally healthy, fish and fruit desserts can be eaten on occasion. However, it is better for persons with more yin cancers to avoid fruit completely —even cooked apples and other more yang fruits. Persons with more yang cancers may occasionally have small amounts but only when craved. On the other hand

---

[12] Plums which have been dried and pickled for many months with sea salt are called *ume* (plum) *boshi* (dry) in Japanese. *Shiso* (beefsteak) leaves are usually added to the plums during pickling to impart a reddish color and natural flavoring. *Umeboshi* plums stimulate the appetite and digestion and aid in maintaining an alkaline blood quality. They are available in many natural food stores.

[13] *Tekka* is literally translated as "iron-fire" (from the Japanese), *tetsu* (iron) and *ka* (fire). This traditional condiment is made from carrot, burdock, and lotus roots which have been finely chopped and sautéed in sesame oil and *miso* for many hours. *Tekka* is usually prepared in a cast iron pan. It is available in many natural food stores.

Table 4   General Yin and Yang Modifications in the Standard Macrobiotic Diet

More yin cancer	Food	More yang cancer
Minimize use of corn.	*Grains*	Avoid buckwheat.
Stronger flavor (more *miso* or *tamari*).	*Soup*	Milder flavor (less *miso* or *tamari*)
Greater emphasis on root varieties (burdock, carrot, turnip, etc.).	*Vegetables*	Greater emphasis on leafy green varieties (*daikon*, carrot, or turnip greens, kale, watercress, etc.).
Stronger seasoning (*miso*, *tamari*, sea salt); slightly heavier cooking.	*Seasoning*	Milder seasoning; more light cooking.
More strongly seasoned; use less often.	*Beans*	More lightly seasoned; may use regularly.
Avoid completely.	*Fruit dessert*	Small amounts of cooked seasonal fruit only when craved.

it is better for persons with more yang cancers to stay away entirely from all animal food, relying only on more lightly cooked vegetable-quality foods. It is also recommended that persons with cancer avoid nuts and nut butters which are very oily and high in protein.

On the whole, the diet should be directed primarily toward restoring the individual's excessively yin or yang condition to one that is less extreme. Once a more neutral, balanced condition has been stabilized, the person's body will no longer need to accumulate toxic excess in the form of cancer. If one keeps this holistic view in mind, one can avoid being caught up in an endless maze of symptoms.

Special Dishes and Considerations

Below are several adjustments which are advisable when preparing and using condiments and other foods:

(1) **Gomashio.** *For more yin cancer*: Prepare 10 to 12 parts roasted sesame seeds to 1 part sea salt. *For more yang cancer*: Prepare with 14 to 16 parts roasted sesame seeds to 1 part sea salt. *For cancers caused by a combination of both*: Prepare with 12 parts seeds to 1 part sea salt. Use about one teaspoonful per day for any type of cancer.

(2) **Roasted Seaweed Powder.** *For more yin cancer*: Approximately 1 teaspoonful per day is recommended. *For more yang cancer*: Slightly less volume is advisable (approximately ½ teaspoonful per day). *For cancers caused by a combination of both*: An in between volume is recommended (½ to 1 teaspoonful per day).

(3) **Umeboshi Plum.** Can be used by persons with all types of cancer. *Umeboshi* plums contain an harmonious balance of more yin factors, such as the natural sourness of the plum, and more yang factors created by the salt, pressure, and aging used in their preparation.

(4) **Tekka.** This more yang condiment can be used by persons with all types of cancer. *For more yin cancer*: Can be used every day (approximately ½ tea-

spoonful). *For more yang cancer*: It is advisable to use a small volume only on occasion.

(5) ***Tamari-Nori* Condiment**. This special condiment, made with *nori* seaweed, can be used to help the body recover its ability to discharge toxic excess. To prepare:

1. Place several sheets of *nori* in water (about ½ cup) and simmer until most of the water cooks down to a thick paste.

2. Add *tamari* soy sauce several minutes before the end of cooking for a light to moderate taste.

This condiment can be eaten by persons with all types of cancer. *Those with more yang cancer* may use a slightly smaller amount (for example ½ teaspoonful per day) while *those with more yin cancer* may use up to 1 teaspoonful per day. *Those with cancers caused by a combination of both* may eat an in between amount.

(6) ***Shio-Kombu* Condiment**. This more yang condiment is very rich in minerals and aids in the discharge of toxins. To prepare:

1. Soak *kombu* until soft and then chop into one-inch square pieces.

2. Add sliced *kombu* (about 1 cup) to ½ cup water and ½ cup of *tamari* soy sauce.

3. Bring to a boil and simmer until the liquid evaporates.

4. Place in a covered jar to keep for several days.

Several pieces of *shio-kombu* may be eaten on a daily basis.

(7) ***Bancha* Tea**. There are now several varieties of *bancha* tea presently available, including green tea, *bancha* twig tea, and *bancha* stem tea. All are produced from the same tea bush. Green tea is harvested in the summer and consists of the green leaves taken from the upper parts of the bush. However, some leaves are left on the plant until fall, at which time they become harder, drier, and brownish in color. These leaves are used to produce the usual *bancha* tea. *Bancha* stem tea is made from the branches and stems of the plant which are dry-roasted. More yin green tea contains much vitamin C and can be used to help offset the toxic effects resulting from the overconsumption of animal foods, while more yang *bancha* stem tea contains less vitamin C but a large amount of minerals. It is advisable for all cancer patients to use the *bancha* tea as their main beverage. However, persons with more yang cancers may occasionally use the green tea for a short duration only. Green tea is not recommended for persons with other types of cancer.

(8) ***Nishime* (Waterless Cooking) Dish**. This special method of preparing vegetables is helpful in restoring strength and vitality to someone who has become physically weak. To prepare:

1. Use a heavy pot with a heavy lid.

2. Soak *kombu* until soft and cut into one-inch square pieces.

3. Place *kombu* in bottom of pot and add just enough water to cover.

4. Add chopped carrots, *daikon*, turnips, or burdock root, lotus root, onions, hard winter squash (acorn or butternut), and cabbage. These should be cut into two inch chunks and layered on top of *kombu*.

5. Sprinkle a small amount of sea salt over the vegetables.

6. Cover and set flame to high until a high steam is generated. Lower flame and cook fifteen to twenty minutes in the high steam. If water evaporates during cooking, add more to the bottom of the pot.

7. When each vegetable has become soft and edible, add *tamari* soy sauce and mix the vegetables by shaking the pot.

8. Replace cover and cook over a low flame for two minutes.

9. Remove cover, turn off flame, and let the vegetables sit for about two minutes, allowing all the steam to escape. There should be no water left in the bottom of the pot.

It is recommended that this dish be included anywhere from two to four times a week.

(9) Steamed Greens Dish. To prepare:

1. Wash and slice the green leafy tops of vegetables such as turnip, *daikon* or carrots. (Kale or watercress may also be used.)

2. Place cut vegetables in a small amount of water at a high boil.

3. Lower flame, cover, and steam for seven minutes.

4. Toward the end, lightly sprinkle *tamari* over the vegetables, and let the dish sit for several minutes.

This dish may be eaten up to once a day with a minimum intake of two times a week.

(10) *Kombu, Azuki* Bean, and Squash Dish. To prepare:

1. Wash and soak one cup of *azuki* beans overnight or for four to six hours.

2. Soak and chop several strips of *kombu* into one-inch square pieces.

3. Place *kombu* in bottom of pot and add beans.

4. Cover with water, bring to a boil, and simmer for thirty minutes until almost soft.

5. Cut hard winter squash (acorn or butternut) into two-inch chunks and place on top of *kombu* and beans. (The amount of squash should be almost equal to the amount of beans.)

6. Sprinkle lightly with sea salt.

7. Cover and cook for another twenty-five to thirty minutes until beans and squash become soft. (If water evaporates, add more from time to time to ensure enough moisture to keep the beans and *kombu* soft.)

8. Add a light amount of *tamari* or sea salt toward the end of cooking.

9. Cover and cook for several more minutes.

10. Turn off the flame and let the dish sit for several minutes before serving.

This dish may be eaten one to three times a week. If squash is not available, carrots may be used instead.

(11) Boiled Salad. To prepare:

1. Wash various greens (kale, dandelion collards, turnip or *daikon* tops, watercress, mustard greens) thoroughly, along with sliced onions, carrots, and green cabbage.

2. Bring several inches of water to a boil and add a pinch of sea salt.

3. Drop vegetables in, several at a time, and boil for one to two minutes.

4. Remove and squeeze out water.

5. Eat as is or with macrobiotic condiments.

Boiled salad may be eaten several times a week in place of raw salad.

(12) *Daikon, Daikon* **Greens, and** *Kombu* **Dish**. To prepare:

1. Wash *daikon* and tops (other hard leafy greens may be used if *daikon* tops are not available).

2. Cut *daikon* into two-inch chunks and place in pot with several pieces of soaked *kombu* on the bottom.

3. Cook for thirty to forty minutes. (Check to make sure that the water does not evaporate.)

4. Add greens.

5. Add *tamari* after several minutes and steam for two to three minutes before serving.

This dish may be eaten several times a week.

(13) *Seitan* **Stew**

Ingredients:

    3 cups of water

    ½ cup of *seitan* cut into one inch pieces (please consult macrobiotic cookbooks for instructions for preparing *seitan*)

    2 pieces (about 18 inches long) of soaked *kombu*

    ½ cup each of three different kinds of roots, cut into one-inch chunks (use onions, carrots, burdock, radishes, *daikon*, turnips, etc.)

    ½ cup each of two kinds of leafy greens, cut into strips (use *daikon* greens, turnip greens, kale, collards, Chinese cabbage, watercress, mustard greens, etc.)

    enough *tamari* for a mildly salty taste

1. Bring water and *kombu* to a boil and simmer for five minutes.

2. Add *seitan* (*tempeh* or *tofu* may be used instead) and boil for two to three minutes.

3. Add root vegetables and boil for five to ten minutes, until the vegetables are tender but still firm.

4. Add greens and *tamari*, cook for two to three minutes, and serve.

This dish may be eaten several times a week, especially by persons who have lost much weight, who have lost their appetite, or who are experiencing weakness. *Mochi* (pounded sweet rice) or white meat fish may be substituted for *seitan* in certain cases.

(14) Sautéed Vegetables. To prepare:

1. Chop carrots, onions, and cabbage very finely.

2. Brush the bottom of the pan with a small amount of sesame oil.

3. When oil becomes hot, add vegetables and sauté for several minutes.

4. Sprinkle in a pinch of sea salt and cover for several minutes.

5. Uncover, season lightly with *tamari*, and cook for two minutes.

6. Turn off flame and serve.

This dish may be eaten several times a week by persons who are allowed some oil. Persons who must avoid the oil may steam or boil their vegetables.

The Importance of Cooking

Macrobiotic cooking is actually very simple once the basic techniques have been mastered. However, before learning the basics, it is very easy to make mistakes, even though various books and publications are consulted. It is very important to attend cooking classes in order to actually see and taste the foods that you wish to prepare. To do this, it is not necessary to spend a great deal of time attending classes. If you are able to learn at least ten or twenty basic dishes, you can go on to develop your own cooking style. Therefore, when beginning macrobiotics, please seek the advice of friends with experience who live near you. Do not hesitate to show them dishes that you have prepared and ask for their advice and suggestions.

One mistake which is common among cancer patients is the overconsumption of flour products. As much as possible, it is better for a cancer patient to eat grains in their whole form rather than in the form of flour. Flour products easily create mucus and intestinal stagnation, and for this reason it is better to avoid items like cookies, muffins, pancakes, and similar foods. Even high-quality macrobiotic bread should be eaten only several times a week and not on a daily basis.[14] It is also advisable for cancer patients to avoid heavily baked or grilled foods.

Way of Life Suggestions

1. You may eat regularly, two to three times a day, provided the proportion is correct and chewing is thorough. Since cancer is a symptom of excess, it is important not to overeat. To prevent this, each mouthful should be thoroughly chewed —at least 100—and preferably 200—times. You may eat as much food as you want provided it is well chewed and thoroughly mixed with saliva, and if you have a tendency to overeat, be sure to get plenty of physical activity. Therefore, if your strength permits, exercise regularly as a part of daily life, including activities like scrubbing floors, cleaning windows, and washing clothes. You may also participate in systematic exercise programs such as yoga, martial arts, or sports.

---

[14] The use of flour has been linked with the occurrence of diarrhea. "Most people have trouble absorbing all-purpose wheat flour, the kind used to make ordinary white bread, and this may be a previously unsuspected cause of diarrhea and other intestinal problems, a study concludes.

"Researchers found that, when people eat white bread, about 20 percent of it is not absorbed into their digestive tracts. The condition is similar to that experienced by some adults who have difficulty digesting milk.

"What it means is that when the average person eats a slice of bread, a fair proportion of it is never absorbed in the small bowel and goes down into the large intestine and can be converted into gas or into stuff that conceivably causes diarrhea, Dr. Michael D. Levitt, one of the researchers, said.

"The study was conducted at the Veterans Administration Medical Center in Minneapolis and published in today's issue of the *New England Journal of Medicine*.

"Using eighteen healthy volunteers, the doctors watched the results when people ate white bread, macaroni, rice bread, or bread made from wheat flour that is low in gluten." (From the *Boston Globe*, April 9, 1981.)

2. Please avoid eating for three hours before going to bed, as food eaten prior to sleeping will stagnate in the body.

3. Do not watch television for an extended period, directly from the front, or at a close distance, so as to minimize your exposure to radiation. Generally, black and white television transmits a weaker form of radiation than color television.

4. Try to avoid wearing synthetic or woolen clothing directly on the skin. Use cotton fabrics as much as possible, especially for undergarments and underwear. If, for example, you must wear nylon stockings for social occasions, remove them as soon as you return. Also, please remove your shoes when you enter your home, so as to allow your feet to breathe and more fully relax. Avoid excessive metallic accessories on the fingers, wrists, and neck. Keep such ornaments as simple and graceful as possible.

5. Go outdoors often in simple clothing, barefoot if possible. Try to walk on the grass, soil, or beach for one-half hour whenever the weather permits.

6. Bring many large green plants into your living room or bedroom to freshen and enrich the oxygen content of the air. As much as possible, keep your windows open to allow fresh air to circulate. Do not keep your home too hot in winter, and try to minimize or avoid air conditioning in the summer.

7. Avoid using electric ranges or cooking devices. Convert to gas at the earliest opportunity. Microwave cooking should also be avoided.

8. Use vegetable quality fabrics—especially cotton—for sheets, pillowcases, and blankets.

9. Scrub your entire body with a hot, wet, squeezed towel every morning and every night before sleeping. Place special emphasis on the hands and fingers, feet and toes.

10. Avoid taking long hot baths or showers unless you have been consuming too much salt or animal food.

11. Try to retire before midnight and get up early every morning.

12. Avoid chemically perfumed cosmetics and soap. For care of the teeth, brush with natural preparations or sea salt.

In general, the patient's environment should be open, happy, and free of any dark or heavy features. This should also extend to such influences as reading material or conversation.

Mental attitude is of course very important. A person with cancer must understand that he or she was responsible for the development of the disease, through his or her diet, manner of thinking and way of life. The patient should be encouraged to reflect deeply, to examine the aspects of his mentality that have produced the problem of cancer and a host of other unhappy situations.

These reflections may also include a review and appreciation of the rich heritage of traditional wisdom developed by many cultures over thousands of years, of the endless wonders of the natural world, including the body's marvellous self-protective and recuperative mechanisms, and of the order of the universe that produces these phenomena.

At the same time, once the decision has been made to reverse the cancer condition by embracing a more balanced approach, the person can forget about the sickness and live as happily, actively, and normally as possible. Cancer patients are often depressed: once the person begins to eat a healthier diet, therefore, he or she needs to be strongly encouraged not to worry and to maintain an optimistic attitude. (For a more thorough discussion of the role of attitude and psychology in both the causation of and the recovery from cancer, please refer to Dr. Northrup's paper in Chapter 2.)

A more complex situation occurs when someone has received chemotherapy or cobalt radiation, or has undergone surgery. In such cases, recovery may be somewhat more difficult but is still quite feasible as long as the patient has normal appetite, good vitality, and the will to live. In a situation such as this, it is particularly vital for both the patient and the members of the family to understand the importance of properly implementing the dietary recommendations. Ideally, they should spend several days (or preferably weeks) learning how to cook properly. They should also seek qualified individual advice on the correct manner of cooking and eating for their particular situation.

Cases that are more serious—so-called terminal cases—require additional attention. In these situations, the cancer may be rapidly spreading and the patient may be in great pain, and his or her appetite may also be diminishing. Such cases require the use of external applications along with the proper way of eating. Food should be cooked to the normal texture and consistency, provided the patient is able to chew and swallow. If the patient has difficulty eating in this manner, it is advisable to mash the foods after they have been cooked. It may also be necessary to cook the food with more water than usual to arrive at a softer, more creamy consistency. Grains, vegetables, beans, and other foods can be cooked in this way and then mashed by hand in a *suribachi*. A blender should not be used for this purpose.

The most important external applications are the *ginger compress, taro potato plaster* and *buckwheat plaster*. The methods for preparing these and their proper uses in cases of cancer are given in the Appendix. Most cancers can be dealt with successfully without the use of external treatments. It is only the 20 to 30 percent that are considered terminal or that have been complicated by previous treatment that require these special methods. The macrobiotic dietary approach can also be combined with these external applications for the relief of a variety of non-cancerous tumors and cysts including brain tumors, fibroid tumors, ovarian cysts, and breast cysts.

In order to further aid in the process of recovery, we also suggest the following daily reflections:

1. Develop your appreciation for nature. Every day, try to set aside several minutes to observe and marvel at the wonder and beauty of our natural surroundings. Appreciate the skies, mountains, sun, wind, rain, snow, and all natural phenomena. Try to regain your sense of marvel at the miracle of life.

2. View everyone you meet with gratitude, beginning with your family and friends, and extend your gratitude to all people.

3. Offer thanks before and after each meal. Express your gratitude to the sun, earth, air, and elements for producing your food, as well as to all those who have grown and prepared it. Use this opportunity to reestablish unity with nature and with society.

The traditional expression, "one grain, ten thousand grains" symbolizes the idea that the earth returns many grains for every one that it receives. A person who is healthy also personifies this ideal in their desire to help others achieve health and happiness.

Therefore, do not hesitate to help other people. Tell them about your experience. As we all know, practically every family is now suffering with cancer, heart disease, or mental illness. If, after you recover, you turn your back on others, it is like hoarding money in a bank account and never using it for your enjoyment. Someone who does this will never become happy, since by helping others, you accelerate your own physical and mental improvement.

When you were born, you never expected to have to sell your time or your life. Exchanging your life for money is not unlike cutting a piece of sausage into slices, weighing, pricing, and offering it to a customer. Please reflect on whether you are really doing what you want to and try to decide how you want to spend the remaining years of your life. If you discover that you are unhappy, begin a process of self-revolution by changing your previous habits and sicknesses into a healthy and sound way of life. With macrobiotics, you can turn your course from one of sickness and decline into one of continuing health and happiness.

We should all realize, in fact, that cancer is not solely the concern of cancer patients and their families. Cancer is merely one dramatic symptom out of many, of the deep misconceptions and ultimately self-destructive tendencies upon which we have built up the grandeur of modern civilization. In a very real sense, cancer is all around us, affecting all of us.

If we can learn to recover from cancer, not by destructive, aggressive, or symptomatic methods, but through a comprehensive reorientation of our very way of life, we may consider that a lasting solution to the multiple ills of society itself may be on the horizon.

Macrobiotics and Heart Disease

Before we can become free of this sickness, or of any illness for that matter, the first thing each of us must do is deeply reflect upon our lives. We must ask ourselves: Is my daily food making my health stronger or is it contributing to my illness? Also, if we are employed in an office in which we spend most of the day sitting at a desk, we need to ask ourselves if there is a balance between our mental and physical activity. Am I living an active, happy life, or is my life sedentary and stagnated?

If we want to be healthy, active, and happy, we need to change our way of eating and seek out more activity.

We know that diet is the underlying cause and the overriding cure of heart disease. Many people with cardiovascular problems have changed their way of eating and activity and have had their health restored. In order to successfully treat heart disease, it is best to reduce the intake of foods high in saturated fat and cholesterol, including red meat, eggs, and dairy products, as well as refined grains, synthetic chemicals, and refined sugar. In their place, it is advisable to eat 50 to 60 percent whole grains (brown rice, wheat, barley, millet, rye, corn, and others); 25 percent locally grown, cooked vegetables and 10 percent beans and sea vegetables. The rest of our diet is made up of fish (if desired), soups (*miso* and *shoyu* broth, particularly), local fruits, some seeds, nuts, and certain condiments. This is the Standard Macrobiotic Diet.

This diet will help the body to discharge toxins and fat deposits that have built up over the years, usually since before a person was a teenager.

Modifications in the Standard Diet

The standard diet can be altered slightly based on an individual's needs and state of health. Basically, there are two types of heart disease. The first is the result of eating foods high in fat and cholesterol leading to hardening of the arteries and fat deposits surrounding the heart. The heart and arteries lose their elasticity and vitality, and the heart labors excessively in order to do its job of pumping blood throughout the body. The fat and cholesterol that collects in the arteries reduce blood and oxygen to the heart and brain. Eventually, enough of these fatty deposits accumulate and cause a heart attack or stroke. This condition, we may say, is very yang—contracted and hardened: the arteries are blocked by fat and cholesterol that has built up.

The second type of heart disease is a condition that arises from drinking too many liquids, particularly alcohol, soda pop, caffeinated beverages and fruit juices and from eating too many refined foods, sugar, and fruits. This type of sickness we can refer to as a more yin condition; the heart is swollen, it beats irregularly, and it is weak.

To treat the more yang, contracted condition, we can begin reducing the foods mentioned earlier, especially foods high in saturated fat and cholesterol. The cooking can be lighter, such as steaming and lightly boiling vegetables. Salads and raw vegetables are fine in moderate amounts as is the occasional use of locally grown fruits and fruit juices such as apple juice or cider. These are examples of good-quality yin foods. Less *miso* and natural *tamari* or *shoyu* may be used in soup which should have a mild flavor. *Wakame* seaweed and some vegetables can also be included in the soup stock.

Beans, especially *azukis*, chickpeas, and lentils, are also encouraged. Hard leafy green vegetables like kale, watercress, and turnip and *daikon* leaves are excellent sources of fiber and very effective in helping the body discharge excess fat which has accumulated in the intestines and elsewhere.

For a yin condition in which the heart is swollen, weak, and beats irregularly, we recommend the Standard Macrobiotic Diet. At the same time, we recommend including more good quality yang foods. The cooking can be longer, and the grains we eat—50 to 60 percent of our daily intake of food—are frequently pressure-cooked. *Miso* soup and *shoyu* broth can be a little stronger, and fish can be eaten as a regular dish. When we eat fish, the portions should be small, and a little grated ginger can be used. Ginger helps digest any oils contained in the dish. Whole grains are always our principal food, even if fish is served with the meal.

Condiments and Special Dishes

For many thousands of years, traditional cultures recognized the importance of natural foods, condiments, and medicines made of natural ingredients. In ancient times, there were no pharmaceutical companies to dispense drugs, so through trial and error and an understanding of nature, ancient people discovered many natural remedies for sickness. Of course, diet is our principal means of preventing and reversing illness. However, traditional people discovered remedies which speed recovery through the utilization of the unique properties of certain plants and food combinations. Many of these remedies were written down in *The Yellow Emperor's Classic of Internal Medicine*, the oldest medical book in the world, in about 2600 B.C. I encourage everyone to read and study this great work.

There are several important medicinal preparations and condiments effective in the therapy of heart disease. For those who suffer from both yang and yin heart conditions, macrobiotic condiments such as *gomashio*, *tekka*, roasted *wakame* seaweed powder, and *umeboshi* plums are very helpful. *Gomashio* has been found to be particularly effective in restoring elasticity to the heart.

For a yang, contracted condition in which a great deal of saturated fat, cholesterol, and salt have been eaten in the past, it is better to use condiments sparingly and increase vegetables such as *daikon* radish, which helps dissolve fat deposits in the arteries and heart. When cooking *daikon*—either boiling or steaming—a few drops of *shoyu* can be used. Scallions and spring onions, used as a garnish or cooked into soups, are also helpful. *Shiitake* mushrooms, used to make a soup stock or cooked in soup, are useful in discharging animal fats. *Kombu* tea, which is *kombu* seaweed boiled in water or *kombu* powder dissolved in boiling water, and pearl barley, if it can be obtained, are both very effective in dissolving fat deposits in the body. Pearl barley can be pressure-cooked or boiled in the same way as other grains or roasted and ground up to be used as a tea with boiling water. Corn is also an excellent grain for strengthening the heart. Watercress and carrot tops cooked together help to restore elasticity to arteries as does *seitan* cooked with a little salt.

Those with a yin, swollen heart can use the condiments mentioned above. In addition, *ranshio* (see Appendix) can be taken once a day for three days—no more. This strengthens the heart and stimulates beating. In traditional Japan—where there was virtually no cardiovascular disease—children would be secretly given *ranshio* by their mothers before a race. It made their hearts stronger and helped them to run better.

Another ancient remedy for a yin condition is *ume-sho-bancha* tea, which also aids in strengthening of the heart. To make this tea, *umeboshi* plum is mixed with *shoyu* and then hot *bancha* tea is added. The order is very important; otherwise, the tea will have little or no effect. (See Appendix.)

Dandelion tea, in which the stem, leaves, and roots of the dandelion (the flower is not used) are mixed with boiling water, can be drunk daily for a yin condition; it is very good for strengthening the heart. *Bancha-shoyu* tea, in which *bancha* twig tea is added to a few drops of natural *shoyu*, creates a more alkaline blood condition, which is fundamental to health.

Blood Quality

When we are healthy, our blood—which is slightly saline—is in an alkaline condition. Fermented products such as *miso* and natural *shoyu* help keep the blood in an alkaline state, thus keeping our overall condition healthy. When we eat such foods as refined sugar, too much fruit or fruit juices, and red meat and dairy products, our blood becomes acidic and the result is that we are prone to more illnesses. Germs thrive in acidic blood.

By eating foods high in saturated fat, artificial chemicals, refined sugar, and other unhealthful substances, other organs, whose job it is to cleanse the blood, are overworked. If we continue to eat this way, the organs are worked to capacity but still cannot fully eliminate such elements from our system. The result is unhealthy blood and weak, tired organs. When our kidneys, liver, spleen, and lungs are unable to cleanse our blood, our hearts suffer all the more. More fat builds up around the heart and the arteries. The heart, like other organs, must labor excessively. You can see that when we are in this condition, our health is quickly declining.

Diagnosing the Heart

The general condition of the heart appears in the tip of the nose. A puffy, swollen nose indicates that the heart muscle is expanded from the excessive intake of more yin foods—sugar, fruit, raw salad, and ice cream—along with the over-consumption of fluid, including alcohol. This condition is often accompanied by a reddish color, caused by the expansion of blood capillaries. The heart and circulatory system are generally overworked and expanded, causing irregularities in the blood pressure and a tendency toward hypertension.

Purple, the most yin of the primary and secondary colors, appears on the tip of the nose usually after many years of overconsuming extremely yin foods and liquids. It is an indication of a dangerous overexpansion of the heart muscle and of the low blood pressure which often results. Persons with this condition face the real possibility of a sudden heart attack.

Many people experience the chronic discharge of oil through the pores on the nose. This is caused by eating too many fatty, sugary, or oily foods and indicates that deposits of fat and cholesterol are accumulating in and around the heart.

A cleft or split in the tip of the nose is a very common sign today. It indicates that the right and left chambers of the heart are not coordinating properly, producing irregular beating or murmuring. This condition is caused by nutritional imbalance, especially a shortage of minerals and complex carbohydrates during the time of the mother's pregnancy. A cleft can also be caused by the excessive intake of more yin simple sugars such as fruits, juices, refined sugars, concentrated sweeteners, and soft drinks, all of which deprive the body of minerals and complex sugars.

Hardness at the tip of the nose is the result of the overintake of saturated fat, especially from animal foods such as meat, poultry, eggs, cheese and other dairy products. Hardening of the arteries, blood vessels, joints, and muscles is indicated, as well as the accumulation of fat around the heart and other more yang, compacted organs like the liver, spleen, kidneys, and prostate gland. If the nose is swollen as well as hard, a heart attack or stroke may occur.

Fig. 11 shows several important areas of the heart. A and B represent the right

Fig. 11   The Heart (Schematic)

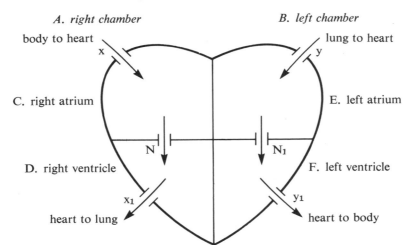

and left chambers of the heart; C and D the right atrium and left ventricle, or upper and lower regions; and E and F the left atrium and ventricle. X and x_1, and y and y_1 represent the flow of blood from the body to the heart and from the heart to the lung on the right side, and from the lung to the heart and the heart back to the body on the left side. N and N_1 represent the valves between the atrium and ventricle of each chamber.

The condition of the heart can also be seen in the entire face (see Fig. 12).

Fig. 12   Diagnosis of the Heart in the Face

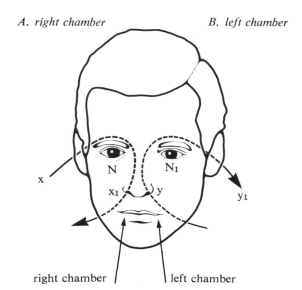

For example, areas A and B correspond to the right and left sides of the face in general. The incoming flow of blood from body to heart, area x, correlates with the canal from the outer right ear in toward the inner ear. The incoming flow of blood from the lung to the heart, area y, correlates with the left nostril and nasal passage. The size of the ear's opening represents the size of that opening to the heart. If mucus or liquid is accumulating in that area of the ear, similar accumulations are taking place in the corresponding area of the heart. Similarly, if mucus occurs in the left nostril or nasal passage, then accumulations are also taking place in the region of the heart which corresponds to area y. The flow of blood from the heart to the lung and from the heart to the body, areas x_1 and y_1, corresponds to the right nasal passage and the left ear canal respectively.

The heart valves, shown above as N and N_1, appear in the eyes. For good, strong heart functions, these valves should be tight and strong; if the eyes become weak and watery, with frequent blinking, then those valves are becoming weak and watery. If the eyes are swollen and red, then some swelling or light inflammation is occurring in the corresponding valves. If the eyes are discharging mucus, then mucus is also accumulating around the valves.

The general condition of areas A and B, the right and left chambers, can be seen in the mouth: if the right side of the mouth is more swollen or loose, this reflects a similar condition in the right chamber. If the mouth as a whole is becoming swollen and loose, the heart is also becoming loose and weak. The activity of the heart can also be determined by the activity of the mouth: a very excitable or talkative person often has an expanded, overactive heart.

It is also possible to judge the coordination of the two chambers by seeing how well the two sides of the mouth coordinate when the person is speaking, as well as by the degree of balance or imbalance of the two sides while the mouth is at rest.

If the face as a whole is bright red or pink, the heart is overworking, usually from too much liquid, sugar, or other more yin foods. If individual capillaries are visible, then the heart is expanded and the person has high blood pressure. If the face is pale, then the heart has become either very tight or very weak, both underactive conditions.

The condition of the heart can also be diagnosed through the hands. The right chamber, area A, appears in the right hand, while region B, the left chamber, appears in the left hand. A reddish color often appears around the periphery of the hand along the thumb and fifth finger area. The flow of blood through both chambers corresponds to this region. In the right hand, the flow of blood from body to heart, area x, corresponds to the tip of the thumb. It then circulates along the periphery of the hand, and continues out along the little finger, which corresponds to area x_1. In the left hand, the flow of blood from lung to heart, area y, corresponds to the tip of the little finger, while the flow from heart to body, area y_1, correlates with the tip of the thumb. (The arrows in Fig. 13 show the direction of blood flow.) Any symptom appearing along this path correlates with

Fig. 13 Diagnosis of the Heart in the Hands

A. right chamber   *B. left chamber*

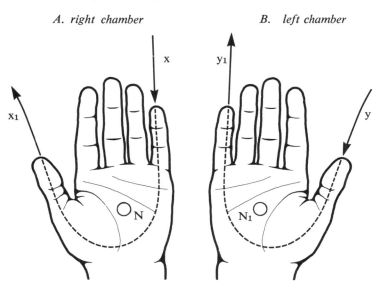

the corresponding region of blood flow in the heart. For example, a chipped or discolored nail on the thumb of the fifth finger or a dark discoloration in the fleshy
part of the thumb indicates stagnations within the flow of blood within the heart.

The condition of the two central valves, marked N and N_1, appears directly in
the center of each palm; if that area is swollen, expanded, or discolored, or if the
person experiences pain when that area is pressed, there exist related troubles with
the corresponding valve such as looseness, weakness, accumulation of fats or
liquid or hardness. If you have the so-called "line of success" which runs straight
down through this area, your valves, N and N_1, are constitutionally strong.

The strength of the grip of each hand generally shows the strength of each
chamber; a comparison of the two hands will show how well the two chambers
of the heart are coordinating and therefore, how efficient the heart's activity is.
In structural terms, if the size, shape, major lines on the palms, and other general
features of the hands are very different, then the two chambers are very different.
In terms of activity, if the two hands are working well together when a person is
using them to do something this also indicates that the two heart chambers are
working well together. If the two chambers are not working together in a smoothly
coordinated, harmonious way, some irregularity of heartbeat will result, and there
will be a tendency for the emotions and the overall character to fluctuate between
extremes, rather than to be consistent, steady, and dependable. Such an imbalanced right or left condition will also be reflected in all the various paired
organs, such as the two kidneys, the two lungs, the liver and spleen, or the two
halves of the brain and sides of the face.

In modern medicine this more holistic view, which considers the interrelation-
ships of the various parts of the body, has been overlooked. Modern anatomy has
measured the size and location of the heart and other organs but has not yet
discovered the overall dynamic function of these organs in relationship to each
other and to the cosmos. One reason for this is that present-day anatomy draws
most of its knowledge from autopsies rather than living organisms. Of course,
when the body is dead, there is not much going on inside besides decay. However,
during a person's life, all of the organs are working in concert with each other.
Thus, in order to strengthen the heart, we need to strengthen the kidneys, liver,
spleen, pancreas, and lungs, since the healthy functioning of the heart depends on
the healthy functioning of our entire system.

The rhythmic beating of the heart is one of nature's most beautiful expressions
of yang and yin, contracting and expanding more than 100,000 times a day, three
billion times in a lifetime.

In the *Gospel According to Thomas*, Jesus says, "If they ask you, 'What is the
sign of your Father in you?' say to them: 'It is a movement and a rest.' " The
heart is a perfect metaphor for the expression of God, the order of the universe,
within each of us. In order to preserve the health of this organ, we must preserve
a balance between yin and yang, between expansion and contraction.

Macrobiotics and the Future World

Recently, a group of leading Japanese engineers and scientists conducted a computer study to determine possible trends of the future. They fed into the computer information covering the last 12,000 years, both from written records and from pre-historic archeological sources. The data covered a wide range of political, economic, scientific, and ideological issues. The computer then arranged this 12,000–year period into twelve unique epochs. The arrangement was as follows:

1. *10000–4000* B.C.   The period of transition from the Stone Age to a premodern form of society.
2. *4000–1000* B.C.   The period of independent small-scale primitive agriculture.
3. *1000* B.C.–A.D. *400*.   The period of more organized agriculture.
4. A.D. *400–1600*.   The period of small-scale cottage industries.
5. A.D. *1600–1900*.   The industrial age, beginning with the Industrial Revolution.
6. *1900–1960*.   The age of automation and mass production.
7. *1960–1980*.   The age of electronics, in which global communication and transportation networks developed.
8. *1980–2000*.   The age of *bionation*.
9. *2000–2010*.   The age of *psychonation*.
10. *2010–2020*.   The age of *para-psychonation*.
11. *2020–2030*.   The age of *ultra-psychonation*.
12. *2033*.   The end of civilization: the computer came to a sudden stop.

All of the investigators involved in this project were puzzled and disturbed when the computer stopped. They rechecked all of their data and again fed it into the computer. Once again, the computer stopped at the year 2033.

From this they concluded that if civilization were to continue in its present direction, some type of world catastrophe or destruction would arise in the near future, through which modern civilization would end. They also concluded that modern society is now moving with very high speed in this direction of self-destruction.

The first seven stages of this process, up to the period of bionation, represent past events which cannot be changed. However, let us consider in more detail the stages which are predicted to occur so as to discover possible approaches for avoiding this conclusion.

The Bionation Age

Bionation refers to the artificial manipulation of or attempt to control natural biological functions, thereby altering the natural quality of an organism. This is achieved through technological intervention. Bionation is not new but has been practiced for many years as a part of modern medicine. It is, however, becoming increasingly widespread and is assuming world-wide proportions.

For example, for many people, modern medicine has recommended the removal of the tonsils and adenoids. However, the tonsils serve an important immunological function, helping to protect the body from more serious degenerative conditions. The removal of the appendix is also a common practice. Although it seems to have no apparent function, the appendix actually aids the entire digestive process, especially in the intestines. Once it has been removed, a person will frequently develop chronic indigestion and gas, as the intestines begin to lose their natural contracting power. Practices such as these contribute to an overall weakening of our natural vitality, including our sexual and reproductive ability, and the intellectual, social, and ideological capacities which depend largely on our physical condition.

Modern medicine also recommends that all children receive a host of immunizations and vaccinations for polio, measles, smallpox, and other illnesses. These vaccinations, however, disturb the natural function of the organism and may contribute to the future development of a more serious disorder such as cancer.

For those who suffer from cancer, heart disease, or some other degenerative disorder, modern medicine will often recommend various surgical procedures in which an organ, gland, or part of an organ is removed and replaced with parts made from plastic or some other artificial material, or with organs from another person. Heart and kidney transplants are now common, while some researchers are pursuing the development and widespread use of totally artificial organs such as the mechanical heart.

The artificial kidney is being used with increasing frequency. Patients with chronic kidney disorders who employ this machine must go to the hospital—in some cases several times a week—for dialysis, during which their blood is cleansed of wastes by passing it through a machine. This treatment is very expensive and once it is started, it must be continued throughout life.

The removal or replacement of body parts has, up until now, been restricted mostly to cases in which the original organ has become diseased. Now, however, one group of researchers has seriously proposed that teenage girls have their breasts removed and replaced with artificial breasts to prevent breast cancer in the future.

The development of the "test tube" baby is also an example of bionation, as is artificial insemination and the manipulation of the DNA, or "genetic material," of the cell. Other examples include the replacement of bones and joints with metal or plastic components, plastic surgery, the use of artificial hearing devices, and the replacement of teeth with metal, plastic, or other materials.

It is surprising how extensive these procedures have become. For example, at a recent macrobiotic conference in Austria, I asked the audience of about 800 people how many had received some type of operation. To everyone's surprise, more than 80 percent responded positively. However, many of us do not realize that the removal or replacement of our organs, glands, and other body parts results in a loss of our genuine human qualities in favor of a more artificial quality. It is not difficult to imagine the replacement of body parts becoming so extensive that, in the near future, the creation of something like Frankenstein will pass from the realm of fiction into reality.

Proceeding with the development of bionation is the effort to replace human beings with a variety of machines. The science of *robotics* deals with this, concentrating on the application of robots to perform many tasks previously carried out by people. Japan is currently the leading manufacturer of robots, with about 14,000 programmable units in operation, followed by the United States which has about 4,100. West Germany, France, Sweden, and the United Kingdom are also using robots for a variety of industrial purposes. The Japanese are also preparing to distribute robots internationally as their next major export item. More extensive uses are also planned for the future; for example, one Japanese electronics firm hopes to be using 100,000 robots in its factories by 1990, while a leading American car manufacturer hopes to install as many as 14,000 by the end of the decade. By the year 2000, literally millions of robots will be in use throughout modern society.

Robots are already replacing humans in tasks such as those performed on assembly lines, but aside from these basic applications, newer generations of robots are now available which can calculate, talk, express emotion, and think independently, as are robots which can produce other robots. In the future, robots may pose the single most important challenge to human beings within industrial society. Unlike humans, robots do not get sick or demand pay raises or vacations. A robot may cost ten, twenty, 100 or 200 thousand dollars to install, but because of its mechanical dependability it will in the long run prove less expensive than human labor. During the twenty-year period of bionation, robots will take over many more jobs in factories, companies, government, and even in management. Along with their use in industry, robots will eventually be available for a variety of other purposes including providing satisfaction for people's emotional and even sexual needs. It is conceivable that someone in the near future will be able to replace their husband or wife with a robot which, unlike its human counterpart, will not suffer from impotence or frigidity, nor argue or become frustrated.

The Psychonation Age

Psychonation refers to the artificial manipulation of and control over the human mind. It is already being practiced throughout the world. For example, many schoolchildren have become hyperactive, due largely to their poor diet, and are difficult to control in the classroom. In many cases, they are sent to psychiatrists who prescribe tranquilizers. Because of their early dependence on drugs, many of these children develop serious drug problems when they get older. Similarly, many patients in mental institutions are heavily drugged in order to keep them under control, while a large number of people practice psychonation on themselves when they take tranquilizers, sedatives, and other over-the-counter drugs.

According to the computer, during the age of psychonation, methods of control such as these may be extended throughout society, with increasing numbers of people having their day-to-day thoughts artificially controlled by outside sources through the administration of drugs and medications.

Further, in order to quell various forms of social unrest such as riots, strikes, or violent crimes, the computer predicts that large population groups may be sedated by putting tranquilizers in city reservoirs or in daily food items like bread. It may also be possible to control the thought processes of an entire population by beaming a certain frequency signal from a satellites or a television transmitting station. In this way, a centralized group or dictatorial power may be able to gain psychological control over an entire country or even the world.

The Para-Psychonation Age

According to the computer, the age of para-psychonation will follow the age of psychonation and will involve the artificial control of fundamental abilities such as extrasensory perception, memory, and future vision, as well as instinctual feelings like love, hope, and sincerity.

The Ultra-Psychonation Age

According to the computer, in the age of ultra-psychonation, ready-made artificial concepts dealing with very basic issues about life, God, and human nature will be imposed upon people. Artificial control may then be extended to all of the most fundamental problems of human life, including intuition, philosophy, and spirituality. As this occurs, everyone will be compelled to think and act in a systematized upon people. Artificial control may then be extended to all of the most fundamental problems of human life, including intuition, philosophy, and spirituality. As this occurs, everyone will be compelled to think and act in a systematized way and to believe that what they are being told is the only real view of life. Meanwhile, robots may take over more than 90 percent of human activities, so that around the year 2033, human civilization as we know it may no longer exist.

The Macrobiotic Alternative

We are presently entering the period of bionation, and many people have already experienced this to one degree or another. If this trend continues, if human beings continue to become increasingly manipulated and mechanized, they will gradually lose their independence and fall more and more under artificial control. If this is extended beyond physical manipulation into the realms of thinking, emotion, and spirituality it will become increasingly difficult, if not impossible, to live as a naturally free human being.

Whether we go in this direction or not largely depends on what happens during the twenty-year age of bionation. If, instead of going toward increasing artificiality, many people choose a more natural method for recovery from cancer, heart disease, and other degenerative disorders, then there is a good possibility that the course of history can be changed. It is our hope that this more natural approach can be widely adopted throughout society and guide the modern health care system in reorienting its priorities toward the elimination of disease at its origin, and not, as is presently the case, merely dealing with symptoms.

What we now refer to as "macrobiotics" is actually the most natural method for achieving this change. By improving the quality of our daily foods, we begin to improve the quality of our blood and body fluids. We can achieve sound physical and psychological health without having to depend on drugs, operations, or other artificial treatments. This improvement in quality begins with one's physical condition and extends to all aspects of life, including judgment, mental qualities, and spirituality. When applied socially, macrobiotics can bring about a future based on the continual development of individual and social health, with all people working toward the goal of a genuinely healthy, productive, and peaceful culture.

Through the remainder of this century many people will choose to go the way of increasing artificiality, believing that technology offers the only valid solution to our modern problems. As a result, they will face increasing degrees of artificial control, with greater competition from robots and the eventual possibility of complete collapse.

Many others, however, will choose another direction as they begin to recover their physical, psychological, and spiritual health as a result of changing their way of life and choosing a more naturally balanced diet. A positive attitude is fundamental to this process, especially as manifested in love and care for others, including parents, ancestors, and offspring, and a sense of wonder and appreciation for nature.

The people who practice this way of life will naturally begin to feel a sense of family unity with each other as a result of eating food of similar quality, which creates a similar physical and mental quality. This family feeling can then naturally develop into a world-wide culture based on mutual love and respect.

Macrobiotics is the inevitable course for all those who wish to maintain their health as well as their independence and individuality. Beginning with the proper selection and preparation of our daily foods, let us secure our endless development toward genuine health, lasting peace, unlimited freedom, and universal love.

External Treatments and Natural Applications

---

1. Ginger Compress

Purpose: Stimulates blood and body fluid circulation; helps loosen and dissolve stagnated toxic matter, cysts, tumors, etc.

Preparation: Place grated ginger in a cheesecloth or cotton sack and squeeze out the ginger juice into a pot of hot water kept just below the boiling point. Dip a towel into the ginger water, wring it out tightly and apply, very hot, directly to the area to be treated. A second, dry towel can be placed on top to reduce heat loss. Apply a fresh hot towel every two to three minutes until skin becomes red.

Special considerations for cancer cases: The ginger compress should be prepared in the usual manner. However, it should be applied for only a short time to activate circulation in the affected area, and should be immediately followed by a taro potato plaster. If ginger compress is applied repeatedly over an extended period, it may accelerate the growth of the cancer, particularly if it is a more yin variety. The ginger compress should be considered only as preparation for the taro plaster in cancer cases, not as an independent treatment, and applied for several minutes only. Please seek more specific recommendations from a qualified macrobiotic advisor.

2. Taro Potato (Albi) Plaster

Purpose: Often used after a ginger compress to collect stagnated toxic matter and draw it out of the body.

Preparation: Pare off potato skin and grate the white interior. Mix with 5 percent grated fresh ginger. Spread this mixture in a half inch thick layer onto a piece of fresh cotton linen and apply the taro side directly to the skin. Change every four hours.

Taro potato can usually be obtained in most major cities in the U.S. and Canada, from Chinese, Armenian or Puerto Rican grocery stores or natural foods stores. The skin of this vegetable is brown and covered with "hair." The taro potato is grown in Hawaii as well as in the Orient. Smaller taro potatoes are the most effective for use in this plaster. If taro is not available, a preparation using regular potato can be substituted. While not as effective as taro, it will still produce a beneficial result. Mix 50 to 60 percent grated potato with 40 to 50 percent grated (crushed) green leafy vegetables, crushing them together in a *suribachi*. Apply as above.

Special considerations for cancer cases: The taro plaster has the effect of drawing cancerous toxins out of the body, and is particularly effective in removing carbon and other minerals which are often contained in tumors. If, when the plaster is removed, the light-colored mixture has become dark or brown, or if the skin where the plaster was applied also takes on a dark color, this change indicates that excessive carbon and other elements are being discharged through the skin. This treatment will gradually reduce the size of the tumor.

If the patient feels chilly from the coolness of the plaster, a hot ginger compress applied for five minutes while changing plasters will help to relieve this. If chill persists, roast sea salt in a skillet, wrap it in a towel, and place it on top of the plaster. Be careful not to let the patient become too hot from this salt application.

3. Buckwheat Plaster
Purpose: Draws retained water and excess fluid from swollen areas of the body.
Preparation: Mix buckwheat flour with enough hot water to form a hard, stiff dough. Apply in a half inch thick layer to the affected area; tie in place with a bandage or piece of cotton linen.
Special considerations for cancer cases: A buckwheat plaster should be applied in cases where a patient develops a swollen abdomen due to retention of fluid. If this fluid is surgically removed, the patient may temporarily feel better, but may suddenly become much worse after several days. It is better to avoid such a drastic procedure.

This plaster can be applied anywhere on the body. In cases where a breast has been removed, for example, the surrounding lymph nodes, the neck, or in some cases the arm, often become swollen after several months. To relieve this condition, apply ginger compresses to the swollen area for about five minutes, then apply a buckwheat plaster; replace every four hours. After removing the plaster, you may notice that fluid is coming out through the skin, or that the swelling is starting to go down. A buckwheat plaster will usually eliminate the swelling after only several applications, or at most after two or three days.

4. Brown Rice Cream: Used to nourish and energize in case of a weakened condition, or when the digestive ability is impaired. Roast brown rice evenly until all the grains turn a yellowish color. To one part rice, add a small amount of sea salt and three to six parts water, and pressure-cook for at least two hours. Squeeze out the creamy part of the cooked rice gruel with a sanitized cheesecloth. Eat with a small volume of condiment, such as *umeboshi* plum, *gomashio* (sesame salt), *tekka*, kelp or other seaweed powder.

5. Carp Plaster: Reduces high fever, as in the case of pneumonia. Crush and mash a whole, live carp, and mix with a small amount of white wheat flour. Spread this mixture onto an oiled paper and apply to the chest. When treating pneumonia, drink one to two teaspoons of carp blood, and then apply the plaster. Take the body temperature every half hour, and immediately remove the carp plaster when the temperature reaches normal.

6. *Daikon* Radish Drink: *Drink No. 1:* Will reduce a fever by inducing sweating. Mix half a cup of grated fresh *daikon* with one tablespoon of *tamari* soy sauce and one quarter teaspoon grated ginger. Pour hot *bancha* tea over this mixture, stir and drink while hot. *Drink No. 2:* To induce urination. Use a piece of cheesecloth to squeeze the juice from the grated *daikon*. Mix two tablespoons of this juice with six tablespoons of hot water to which a pinch of sea salt has been added. Boil this mixture and drink only once a day. Do not use this concoction more than three consecutive days without proper supervision and never use it without first boiling.

7. *Dentie* (*Denshi*): Prevents tooth problems, promotes a healthy condition in the mouth and stops bleeding anywhere in the body by contracting expanded blood capillaries. Bake an eggplant, particularly the calix or cap, until black. Crush into a powder and mix with 30 to 50 percent roasted sea salt. Use daily as a tooth powder or apply to any bleeding area—even inside the nostrils in cases of nosebleed—by inserting wet tissue dipped in *dentie* into the nostril.

8. Dried *Daikon* Leaves: Used to warm the body and to treat various disorders of the skin and female sexual organs. Also helpful in drawing odors and excessive oils from the body. Dry fresh *daikon* leaves in the house, away from direct sunlight, until they turn brown and brittle. (If *daikon* leaves are unavailable, turnip greens can be substituted.) Boil four to five bunches of the leaves in four to five quarts of water until the water turns brown. Stir in a handful of sea salt and use in one of the following ways:

1. Dip cotton linen into the hot liquid and wring lightly. Apply to the affected area repeatedly, until the skin becomes completely red.
2. Soak in a hot bath in which this mixture has been added.
3. Women experiencing problems in their sexual organs should sit in the bath described above with the water at waist level, the upper portion of the body covered with a towel. Remain in the water until the whole body becomes warm and sweating begins. This generally takes about ten minutes. Repeat as needed, up to ten days.
4. Strain the liquid and use as a douche to eliminate mucus and fat accumulations in the uterine and vaginal regions. This douche can be used after the hot bath described above or by itself.

9. Ginger Sesame Oil: Activates the functions of the blood capillaries, circulation, and nerve reactions. Also relieves aches and pains. Mix grated fresh ginger with an equal amount of sesame oil. Dip cotton linen into this mixture and rub briskly into the skin of the affected area.

10. Grated *Daikon*: A digestive aid, especially for fatty, oily, heavy foods, and for animal food. Grate fresh *daikon* (red radish or turnip can be used if *daikon* is not available). Sprinkle with *tamari* soy sauce and eat about a tablespoonful.

11. Scallion, Onion, or *Daikon* Juice: Will neutralize the poison of a beesting or an insect bite. Cut either a scallion, onion or *daikon*, or their greens, and squeeze out the juice. (If you cannot obtain these vegetables, red radish can be used.) Rub the juice thoroughly into the wound.

12. *Kuzu* Drink: Strengthens digestion, increases vitality and relieves general fatigue. Dissolve a heaping teaspoon of *kuzu* powder into one cup of cold water. Bring the mixture to a boil, reduce the heat to the simmering point and stir constantly until the liquid becomes a transparent gelatin. Now stir in one teaspoon of *tamari* soy sauce and drink while hot.

13. Lotus Root Plaster: Draws stagnated mucus from the sinuses, nose, throat and bronchi. Mix grated fresh lotus root with 10 to 15 percent pastry flour and 5 percent grated fresh ginger. Spread a half-inch layer onto cotton linen and apply the lotus root directly to the skin. Keep on for several hours or overnight, and repeat daily for several days. A ginger compress can be applied before this application to stimulate circulation and to loosen mucus in the area you are treating.

14. Mustard Plaster: Stimulates blood and body fluid circulation and loosens stagnation. Add hot water to dry mustard and stir well. Spread this mixture onto a paper towel, and sandwich it between two thick cotton towels. Apply this "sandwich" until the skin becomes red and warm, and then remove.

15. *Ranshio*: Used to strengthen the heart, and to stimulate heartbeat and blood circulation. Crush a raw egg and mix with one tablespoon of *tamari* soy sauce. Drink slowly. Use only once a day and for no more than three days.

16. Raw Brown Rice and Seeds: Will eliminate worms of various types. Skip breakfast and lunch. Then, on an empty stomach, eat a handful of raw brown rice with a half-handful of raw seeds such as pumpkin or sunflower seeds, and another half-handful of chopped raw onion, scallion or garlic. Chew everything very well, and have your regular meal later in the day. Repeat for two to three days.

17. Salt *Bancha* Tea: Used to loosen stagnation in the nasal cavity or to cleanse the vaginal region. Add enough salt to warm *bancha* tea (body temperature) to make it just a little less salty than seawater. Use the liquid to wash deep inside the nasal cavity through the nostrils, or as a douche. Salt *bancha* tea can also be used as a wash for problems with the eyes.

18. Salt Pack: Used to warm any part of the body. For relief of diarrhea, for example, apply the pack to the abdominal region. Roast salt in a dry pan until hot and then wrap in a thick cotton linen or towel. Apply to the troubled area and change when the pack begins to cool.

19. Salt Water: Cold salt water will contract the skin in the case of burns, while warm salt water can be used to clean the rectum, colon and vagina. When the skin is damaged by fire, immediately soak the burned area in cold salt water until irritation disappears. Then apply vegetable oil to seal the wound from the air. For constipation or mucus and fat accumulations in the rectum, colon, and vaginal regions, use warm salt water (body temperature) as an enema or douche.

20. Sesame Oil: Use to relieve stagnated bowels or to eliminate retained water. Take one to two tablespoons of raw sesame oil on an empty stomach to induce the discharge of stagnated bowels. To eliminate water retention in the eyes, put a drop or two of pure sesame oil in the eyes with an eyedropper, preferably before sleeping. Continue up to a week, until the eyes improve. Before using the sesame oil for this purpose, boil and then strain it with a sanitized cheesecloth to remove impurities.

21. *Tamari Bancha* Tea: Neutralizes an acidic blood condition, promotes blood circulation and relieves fatigue. Pour one cup of hot *bancha* twig tea over one to two teaspoons of *tamari* soy sauce. Stir and drink hot.

22. *Tofu* Plaster: Is more effective than an ice pack to draw out a fever. Squeeze the water from the *tofu*, mash it and then add 10 to 20 percent pastry flour and 5 percent grated ginger. Mix the ingredients and apply directly to the skin. Change every two to three hours.

23. *Umeboshi* Plum; Baked *Umeboshi* Plum; Powdered, Baked *Umeboshi* Plum Pit: Neutralizes an acidic condition and relieves intestinal problems, including those caused by microorganisms. Take two or three *umeboshi* plums with *bancha* twig tea. Or, you may bake the plums or their pits until black. If you are using the pits, powder them and add a tablespoonful to a little hot water or tea.

24. *Ume-Sho-Bancha*: Strengthens the blood and the circulation through the regulation of digestion. Pour one cup of *bancha* tea over the meat of one-half to one *umeboshi* plum and one teaspoon of *tamari* soy sauce. Stir and drink hot.

25. *Ume-Sho-Kuzu* **Drink**: Strengthens digestion, revitalizes energy and regulates the intestinal condition. Prepare the *kuzu* drink according to the instructions in Number 12, and add the meat of one-half to one *umeboshi* plum along with the soy sauce. An eighth of a teaspoon of grated fresh ginger may also be added.

Special Note: It is generally advisable to use the above special preparations under the guidance of a qualified macrobiotic advisor.

Chapter 2

Cancer and Diet

Common Cancer Myths

Christiane Northrup, M.D.

From the time I first walked onto a cancer ward as a medical student, and participated in orthodox therapies for the disease, I have persisted in feeling that these treatments were often inadequate at best and harmful at worst. At that time, the fields of cancer chemotherapy and radiation therapy were relatively new. Many of the drugs and radiation treatments were given via experimental "protocols," in an attempt to determine which combinations would yield the best survival results in given tumor types. A certain body of knowledge has been gained from this approach, but often the price of a "cure" or palliation is too high.

Cancer now kills one in five people in the U.S. It is the major cause of death in children (excluding accidents) and middle-aged women. One in eleven American women can expect to get breast cancer, for which the survival rate has not appreciably changed in forty years. The annual number of deaths from cancer is approaching 300,000. In the next decade one in four people will die of the disease if present trends continue.

The Orthodox View of Cancer

The orthodox approach to the nature of cancer is well-summarized by Cornelius Moerman, a Dutch physician specializing in nutritional cancer therapies: "No one in the world knows what cancer is, although almost all physicians have become accustomed to speaking of cancer by saying, 'This is cancer, this is not,' instead of 'We call this cancer and we do not call that cancer,' thus causing the serious delusion, especially in the minds of the general public, that it is known exactly what cancer is." Seventy-five years ago, when cancer research first started on a broad scale, the situation was the same. But in order to start research on something, you must have a definition of what it is. A group of scholars, therefore, drew up a preliminary outline called "The Cellular Hypothesis" based on the following observations of cancer:

1. Cancer is a local disease.
2. The disease consists of the formation of tumors.
3. The tumor is made up of abnormally-formed cells.
4. These cells are growing independently and their growth cannot be halted.

This hypothesis, according to Moerman, has never been scientifically validated. But as time went on, it was forgotten that all cancer research, in those days and today, was founded on this hypothesis. Therefore, the treatment of cancer by operations, radiation and drugs can never be considered scientific treatment.

This discrepancy has been hidden by the custom of speaking of the "generally accepted view," until we have gradually lost sight of the fact that behind this "generally accepted view" an enormous blunder lies hidden.

Orthodoxy today considers cancer to be a number of tumor diseases with multiple causes and varying treatments—some 270 separate tumors, in fact, with countless manifestations. Without knowing what cancer actually is, in other words, treatment is based solely on what is *seen*. The very name *oncology* comes from the Greek *onkos*, meaning lump or tumor. All the major medical and surgical disciplines now have cancer subspecialties within them, such as gynecologic oncology, pediatric oncology, medical oncology, and so on. Much controversy exists among these subspecialties as to what constitutes optimal treatment for a particular cancer, and as to how statistics should be compiled and reported.

Moerman puts it succinctly when he says, "The great variety of theories on cancer, which are forever contradicting each other and competing amongst each other, are a clear indication of the fact that cancer is nothing but a name for something that is shrouded in mystery."

The Orthodox Approach to Treatment

Until very recently, the entire energy of oncology has gone into the development of ways to remove, reduce, poison, or burn out tumors: the idea being that the shrinking of a tumor equals a cure. The orthodox concept of cancer cures also involves the "five year survival" concept. This means that if a person who has had cancer is free of symptoms and obvious recurrences over a five-year period, then he is cured. A slow growing or latent cancer appearing or reappearing in the first hour of the first day of the sixth year following treatment does not fall from the statistics.

There is another problem with survival statistics: if a patient dies of complications from the treatment itself, such as overwhelming infection from the effects of chemotherapy, the cause of death is listed as infection, not as cancer. Only the surgical removal of a small primary tumor in which no metastases have occurred and when many years of symptom free life have passed, or only those tragically few cases where chemotherapy and radiation do seem to have suppressed all tumor activity without recurrence—only these cases fall anywhere close to the real meaning of "cure."

Furthermore, since the diagnosis of cancer is made on the basis of microscopic sections of tissue, it is clear that unless one microscopically sectioned the enitre body, one could not be really sure of a total cancer cure. The five-year survival rate has not held up too well in many cancer types, and in fact has virtually been abandonded for breast cancer. In one British study of women under the age of thirty who had microscopic foci of breast cancer removed, it was found that twenty-five years later 80 percent had died of their original disease, despite the fact that their original tumors had been tiny and had been completely removed.

Causes of Cancer

The many theories about what causes cancer simply add to the general confusion surrounding the disease. One of the best known factors cited as causing cancer is *radiation*. Radiation can of course cause mutations in cells, which can in turn reproduce and lead to cancer. This is evidenced by the high rate of leukemia in Hiroshima victims, and by the higher rate of thyroid cancer in those adults whose thymus glands were radiated as children; radiologists also have a higher rate of leukemia than all other medical professions. Many people, though, are exposed to continually high levels of radiation and remain healthy, while many of those exposed only to low levels get cancer.

The same can be said of *carcinogens* (such as asbestos or coal tar), substances known to produce cancer by affecting the organism's genetic information over a period of time. It is well-known that the incidence of cancer increase markedly with increasing industrialization and environmental pollution. A counterargument here is that better medical care in industrialized countries allows more people to live long enough to get cancer. Some medical authorities, in fact, believe that all of us would get cancer if we only lived long enough! And yet in some parts of the world, for example in Tibet, where people often live over 100 years, cancer is almost unknown. So, although there is no simple cause and effect relationship between carcinogens, radiation or old age and cancer, there is clearly a broad statistical correlation. But this does not explain why some people who have smoked for forty years, for example, do not get lung cancer, while some who do not smoke at all do.

This brings us to the idea of a *genetic predisposition* to cancer. It is clear, for example, that certain families are highly susceptible to the disease. Furthermore, special strains of laboratory animals have been bred, 80 percent of which get cancer. Because Japanese women have one of the lowest cancer rates in the world (especially for breast cancer), it was felt until recently that they had an inherent racial resistance. But now we know that Japanese women living in this country for ten years or more have a breast cancer rate equal to that of U.S. women; and we know that for those Japanese women living in Hawaii, where the culture and diet are halfway between that of the U.S. and that of Japan, the breast cancer rate is twice that of Japan and half that of the U.S.

An experiment done by Dr. Vernon Riley at the University of Washington with cancer prone mice casts further doubt on the genetic theory. He was working with two groups of mice, all of which had an 80 percent chance of contracting breast cancer. One group was exposed to a very stressful environment, the other to one that was stress-free. At the end of the study, 97 percent of the stressed rats had breast cancer, compared to only 7 percent of those in the stress-free group. So although genetics plays some role in cancer production, further explanation is needed.

Because the most outstanding successes in orthodox medicine have been in the treatment of infectious diseases with antibiotics, it makes sense that drug-oriented conventional medicine would try to fit cancer into an infectious disease model by looking for a *viral* etiology. The link between herpes type II virus and cancer of the cervix has been widely publicized as an example, but the evidence is not very convincing. Viruses are often found in tumors, but it is not clear whether the virus is there because of the weakened tissue in the tumor or as a causative agent of the tumor. The following are some of the problems with the virus theory:

1. Viruses and other microbiological elements live in symbiosis with the human organism, usually not causing disease unless the host is compromised.
2. Every living healthy being carries these microscopic elements; they are even found in the blood of healthy newborns.
3. When an injection of living cancer cells and virus is given to a healthy organism, nothing happens because the immune system kills the invaders. (More about the immune system later.)

Diet and Psychology

The evidence linking cancer and diet is mounting daily. Including diet as a possible cause of cancer is a relatively recent phenomenon in orthodox medicine. Studies have shown, for example, that decreased caloric intake is associated with decreased incidence of cancer. It follows that an increased caloric intake is associated with increased incidence of cancer. Dr. Denis Burkitt's studies linking high dietary fiber with very low rates of colonic cancer have prompted many Western physicians to prescribe bran in their patients' diets, since bowel cancer is very common in the U.S.

In the book *Cancer: A Manual for Practitioners*, published by the Massachusetts Division of the American Cancer Society, Blake Cady, M.D. states that the "enormous reduction in death rates seen in the Mormons and the Seventh-Day Adventists, who are abstentious and diet-conscious, far outweigh the effects of our current medical care and are far cheaper than our massive halfway medical technology." Interestingly, Max Gerson, M.D. was branded as a heretic twenty years ago for making a connection between diet and cancer, and for treating via nutrition alone.

Along with the role of nutrition, one of the most exciting factors being studied in relation to cancer is the *psychological* component. The link between emotions and illness has been known for centuries. As far back as 537 B.C., the ancient and respected physician Galen noted that women who were depressed and melancholy were more apt to get breast cancer than cheerful ones. But in recent times, the study of the mind and of the body has been split into separate disciplines, often resulting in a lack of communication and acknowledgment of this important aspect of medicine.

In a classic study of 100 cancer patients by Dr. Oleta Evans in 1926, entitled "A Psychological Study of Cancer," it was found that grief due to the loss of a significant relationship was the most common predisposing cause in cancer. Dr. Lawrence LeShan, a psychologist, found in a controlled study of 500 cancer patients the following psychological pattern: childhood isolation and despair, poor parental relationships, establishment in adult life of a strong relationship or job into which much energy was poured, subsequent loss of this relationship or job through death, divorce or retirement, leading to the same emotions and feelings as in childhood. Within six to eight months of the loss, the terminal cancer appeared. Out of LeShan's 500 patients, 76 percent demonstrated this pattern, versus only 10 percent among the controls.

The work of Dr. Carl Simonton confirms the concept of a *cancer prone personality*. His work at the Cancer Counseling Research Center in Fort Worth, Texas, incorporates this information into a unique treatment program. During training as a radiation oncologist, Simonton became very interested in why two patients, both with the same disease, would react so differently, some recovering their health and others dying almost immediately. The difference seemed to be that those who lived despite their prognosis felt they exerted some *control* over their illness while the other group felt fairly helpless. The cancer patient often sees himself as a victim and is unable to handle stress properly. Of course, feelings of helplessness and hopelessness do not cause cancer, but they do seem to create a climate for the disease to develop by interfering with the *immune system*.

The work of Dr. Hans Selye has been instrumental in showing the physiologic mechanisms by which stress, sadness, etc., can decrease immune functioning. Simonton's work tends to mobilize the patient's immune system by using stress alteration techniques as an adjunct to routine cancer therapy, and he brings out the patient's own volition in the healing process. (See Figs. 14 and 15 for Simonton's theories of disease development and recovery.)

To many involved in the holistic approach to disease, mental attitude is clearly acknowledged as constituting as much as half or more of the overall program. The patient must realize that he is responsible for helping to treat his cancer. Those with the passive attitude of "the doctor will do this for me" are not appropriate subjects for this approach.

The Immune System

The link between all of the proposed mechanisms involved in cancer production is the immune system. The growing field of immunology, which not long ago was considered outside the pale, has now become an area of intense research. Clearly any part of an explanation concerning cancer must ultimately deal with *the suppression of the body's natural defenses* against disease.

This is not a new theory. In the 1920's, James Beard, a Scottish embryologist, speculated that due to their overriding similarities, the *trophoblast* cell (normally present only during pregnancy as part of the embryo and placenta) and the cancer cell are actually one and the same. But when trophoblast, a cell which has the potential to become any part of the body, occurs outside of the uterus, it is cancer —trophoblast at the wrong place and time. Many researchers today feel that breakthroughs in cancer will come by studying the placenta and fetus, and by learning how a pregnant woman manages to nurture foreign tissue in her body without rejecting it.

Erlich's hypothesis of the early 1900's postulated that the body recognizes cancer as "not-self" and can mount an antibody defense. This theory has often been proved, but cancer patients seem to have "blocking proteins" that keep their antibodies from recognizing and destroying the tumor cells.

Immune theory helps to explain many of the side effects of traditional cancer therapy. Chemotherapy and radiation, both meant to poison the tumor locally, actually destroy both the cancer and the patient at the same time. Because they are non-specific in their action, they potentially harm all the cells, and especially the fast growing ones such as the bone marrow, where the white blood cells of the immune system are produced, thus leaving the defense mechanisms paralyzed. We are finding that some of these modalities actually increase the patient's chances of getting other cancers (if they live long enough). Clearly, orthodox therapies are needed in life-threatening situations, such as when a tumor is encroaching upon the vital organs (e.g., the heart or spinal column). But it is time we incorporated more holistic nutritional and psychological approaches into our treatment, so that if one chooses to employ conventional therapies, one could bolster the immune system and lessen the side effects. Some clinics are in fact now doing this, with quite good success. Clearly, any concept of a cancer cure needs an efficiently functioning immune system.

Fig. 14 Mind/Body Model of Cancer Development
(Simonton, et al., *Getting Well Again*, St. Martin's Press, New York, 1978)

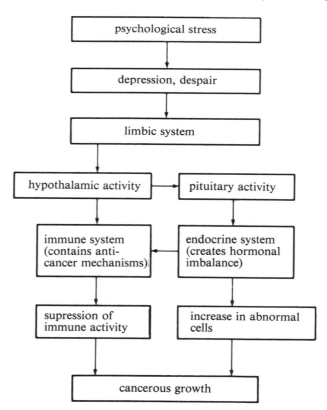

Holistic Approaches

Because of the failure of orthodox modalities to stem the incidence of and suffering from cancer, more and more people are turning to unorthodox approaches with fresh interest. *Holism* views cancer and all degenerative diseases as deficiency states. Cancer is viewed as a chronic systematic metabolic disease characterized by a breakdown of the body's natural functions as a result of deficiency and dysfunction, not directly related to pathogens. Numerous outside factors help to organize but do not cause the condition. The induction of cancer would be impossible without the accompanying weakening of the basic body chemistry and immune system. So the tumors themselves are just *symptoms* of the disease state, and not the disease itself. Hence, the treatment of symptoms, however vital in life-threatening situations, is by no means a treatment of the disease. Only a treatment program which takes into account the entire metabolism can adequately cope with the disease. Thus, most holistic therapies postulate that all degenerative disease is susceptible to management by dietary means. The approaches are some-

Fig. 15 Mind/Body Model of Recovery
(same source as Fig. 14)

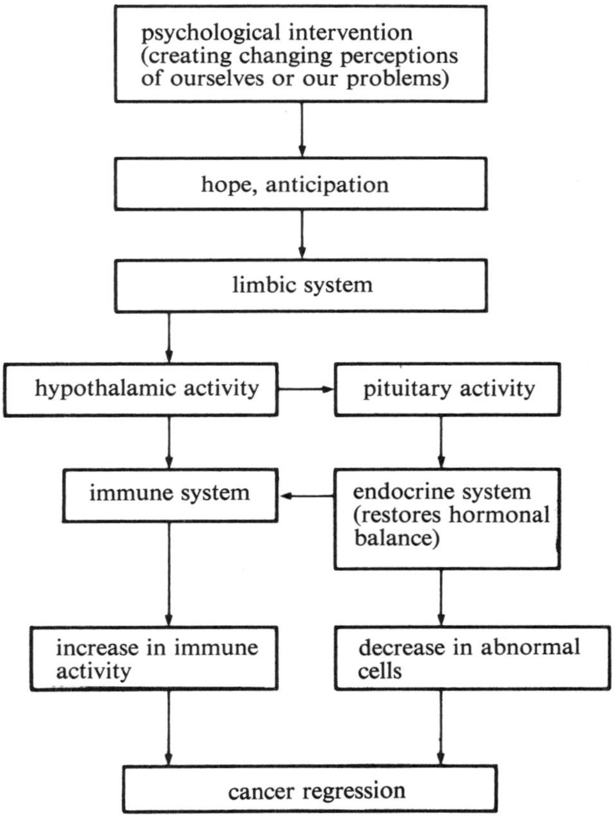

```
        ┌──────────────────────────────────┐
        │ psychological intervention       │
        │ (creating changing perceptions   │
        │ of ourselves or our problems)    │
        └──────────────────────────────────┘
                        │
        ┌──────────────────────────────────┐
        │         hope, anticipation       │
        └──────────────────────────────────┘
                        │
        ┌──────────────────────────────────┐
        │          limbic system           │
        └──────────────────────────────────┘
                        │
        ┌────────────────────┐      ┌────────────────────┐
        │ hypothalamic       │─────▶│ pituitary activity │
        │ activity           │      └────────────────────┘
        └────────────────────┘                │
                │                    ┌────────────────────┐
        ┌────────────────────┐      │ endocrine system   │
        │ immune system      │◀─────│ (restores hormonal │
        └────────────────────┘      │ balance)           │
                │                    └────────────────────┘
                │                             │
        ┌────────────────────┐      ┌────────────────────┐
        │ increase in immune │      │ decrease in        │
        │ activity           │      │ abnormal cells     │
        └────────────────────┘      └────────────────────┘
                │                             │
        ┌──────────────────────────────────┐
        │         cancer regression        │
        └──────────────────────────────────┘
```

what varied, but all involve abstinence from meat and increased consumption of whole foods, as well as major life-style changes.

The data on holistic approaches to cancer is necessarily clouded by the fact that the vast majority of cancer patients turn to macrobiotics and other alternative methods only after having exhausted the full gamut of orthodox modalities. Their immune systems are often lethally depressed, and past therapy and/or cancer may have done much irreparable damage. These factors greatly influence the course of nutritional therapy. Another problem is that of a control group: the holistic practitioner would consider it unethical to deny some people treatment on a random basis for study purposes.

Moreover, under the normal treatment and measurement protocols of standard oncology, there are no parameters for measuring the success of holistic medicine in cancer control, because the conventional parameters are limited to what happens or what does not happen to the tumor. Holistic medicine, however, is not concerned with the tumor per se—it is concerned with how the patient feels as a whole; rarely does a patient die of cancer feeling really well.

Happily, with increasing research and consumer pressure, orthodox medicine is slowly changing its attitude. In the book *Clinical Oncology: A Multidisciplinary Approach* (the standard text on the subject used by medical students), Dr. Roger Terry states, "It is important to recognize that the disease we call cancer is determined more by the ever-changing reactive state of the individual host who harbors the tumor than by the histologic characteristics of the cancer cells in that host. Cancer should never be looked upon as a disease entity, but only as a traditional term which describes a neoplastic process. Many cancers could be prevented by utilizing the readily accessible knowledge that has accumulated."

And Blake Cady, M.D., in his introduction to *Cancer: A Manual for Practitioners*, states that "progress in clinical cancer control will certainly not be achieved by some specific breakthrough from the research laboratory."

He goes on to say that "the public has a major role in the control of cancer, through curbing such destructive habits as smoking and inappropriate diet. The public must also realize that a number of experts are increasingly convinced that the medical profession may have only a limited role in disease control. In developed countries the individual's health is now largely in his own hands. He can do more to preserve his health and extend his life by controlling his own behavior than he can by making full use of all the specific preventive or therapeutic services available to him."

I could not agree more.

Addendum

Since my introduction to macrobiotics and the writing of the foregoing piece, I have gained a much broader experience with this way of life and healing both in my personal and family life and through observing a growing number of patients who are using this approach with various illnesses. The thing that impressed me most when I first learned about macrobiotics was the way people's faces changed while eating this way. It was and continues to be astounding to see cancer patients and those with other serious illnesses who look (and feel) ten years younger after several months on this diet. Such rejuvenating benefits from standard medical therapy are rare indeed. Because of this and my lifelong interest in holistic medicine, I have continued my study of macrobiotics while at the same time practicing obstetrics and gynecology along fairly traditional lines.

I would like to share the following thoughts about healing in general and macrobiotics in particular:

1. The most important aspect in recovering from one's illness is a positive mental attitude. If one's attitude remains that of a helpless victim denying any role in the onset of the disease, then there will seldom be a cure. One must also believe in one's ability to help himself.

2. If at some level a person does not truly desire to regain health, it is useless to force him or her to try a healing modality such as macrobiotics. No amount of pressure from family or friends will help. It is better to gently support the ill person in the therapy of his or her choice—including all traditional modalities— while at the same time helping that person to discover his or her inner healing resources.

3. When one starts macrobiotics it is important not to reject standard Western medicine completely. There are times when the traditional approach can be extremely helpful and even lifesaving. The point is to understand its limitations. And the same is true of any healing modality, including macrobiotics. A Caesarian section in a hospital setting has the potential to be as *holistic* as a home birth.

4. Family support is crucial. Without some type of support within one's immediate family or circle of friends it is extremely difficult to practice the macrobiotic diet in the Western world at this time, particularly if one is ill. With support, however, it becomes an exciting adventure.

5. For optimum results when changing one's diet, I would highly recommend a personal counseling session with a qualified macrobiotic advisor. Some of the adverse outcomes from so-called macrobiotics in the past could have been prevented through more adequate knowledge of macrobiotic dietary principles.

6. I am convinced by my experience to date that when practiced with a sense of humor and common sense, macrobiotics is an excellent dietary approach for anyone who desires optimal health and ideally should be started *before* one becomes ill. In fact, after eating this way for a time, all desire to return to former ways of eating disappears. There is never a sense of deprivation. The diet is varied enough to satisfy anyone's taste once health has been regained.

Macrobiotics should not be viewed, then, as a diet to be followed for a month or two only to be stopped once one is "cured." To be truly macrobiotic in the broadest sense is a goal which will take most of us years to reach. More than a style of eating, macrobiotics is a philosophy based on universal principles. But eating this way is a crucial first step toward true health and understanding.

Macrobiotics, Cancer, and Medical Practice

Keith Block, M.D., Penny Block M.A.

To the modern public, the approach that Dr. Block recommends might sound new and exotic. Actually it is age-old. The staple foods of macrobiotics have been eaten traditionally around the world: brown rice, millet, barely, oats, rye, wheat, corn, and buckwheat. In our practice, the approximate quantities of a basic diet are: 50 percent cooked whole grains; 25 percent fresh, local vegetables; 15 percent beans and sea vegetables; and about 10 percent fish, soup, condiments, fruits, seeds, and nuts. Of course, it is necessary to modify this food plan for each individual. (See Chapter 1.)

People having heard about macrobiotics frequently come with a harvest of questions. The public wants to know, "What foods do I need to eat? Where do I purchase them? How do I prepare them?" Cancer patients and their families— a devoted granddaughter trekking 100 miles to Evanston to gather information; the mother of a nine-year-old cancer victim; the husband of a twenty-nine-year-old with a colon malignancy—all are hunting for explanations. At the same time, they are positive in their readiness to pursue a dietary solution to one of modern life's most dread diseases. "What" and "how" are usually ice-breakers before the paramount question surfaces: "Dr. Block, from a medical perspective, why do you think macrobiotics works?"

The marvel is—it does work. And not only for cancer patients. In his practice, Dr. Block has successfully treated people with many afflictions. For John, a strapping thirty-three-year-old suffering from high blood pressure, impotence was the rueful side-effect of his prescribed medication. He was amazed that six weeks of macrobiotic eating enabled him to discontinue his drugs comfortably. Up until then, John had resigned himself to a permanent dependence on anti-hypertensives.

It seemed almost miraculous to Jim, a twenty-two-year-old diabetic, that within only three weeks on a macrobiotic regimen, he safely whittled his insulin doses down to less than half of the original prescription. Nighttime shots were called to a halt. For Jim this meant abandoning his former eating style. However, he was so pleased with his rapid improvement that he hardly regretted giving up his old food habits. Even diabetic specialists at the famed Joslin Clinic were blinking their eyes in amazement at the swift results of Jim's diet. Medical professionals at the clinic supported Jim in his eating strategy, after analyzing it carefully. One foresaw that in the coming years all diabetic treatment would rely on a dietary therapy like Jim's.

For five years, Jeanine, a woman in her early forties had suffered with a urinary tract infection. During this time she had gone to a dozen different G.U. specialists.

None of the seventeen medications they had prescribed had offered her relief. Not surprisingly, she was growing despondent. When she visited, Dr. Block advised her to stop the medications and begin a basic macrobiotic diet. Due to her specific condition, however, he recommended that she temporarily eliminate fruits, oils, and flour products. One week later, her chronic infection had disappeared; and it did not reappear. Her words practically skipped along the telephone wire when she called to announce triumphantly, "For the first time in fifteen years, I am free of this pesky disorder."

Jeanine's jubilance is representative of many who conscientiously follow their food plans. Relief from illness is not the reward of only a few showcase examples. In the vast experience of Michio Kushi, president of the East West Foundation and author of *The Book of Macrobiotics*, any disorder can find remedy in the macrobiotic diet. From glaucoma to asthma, from herpes to colitis, the results of eating correctly are astonishing.

However, it is cancer which looms as the dread affliction of modern society. One patient confided to Dr. Block that no judge could have delivered a more devastating sentence than the oncologist's words, "terminal cancer." Particularly at night, this patient was haunted by relentless and horrifying images of cancerous growths boring through his body tissue and painfully consuming his life.

Cancer has become epidemic in proportion. According to the American Cancer Society, more than fifty-five million Americans now living will have cancer in their lifetimes. It will strike two out of every three families. This could mean that if everyone in your family survives free of cancer, possibly the family living across the hall from you, and another family in the downstairs apartment will lose to cancer. A medical estimate is that by the year 2000, every other person will be stricken with cancer. Of cancer cases, two-thirds are declared incurable. The statistics are staggering and unavoidable. Eleven hundred people per day, one person every eighty seconds is dying in this country of cancer.

Open your newspaper tomorrow and chances are you will read of another household substance, industrial compound, cosmetic ingredient, or even familiar over-the-counter analgesic which has been indicted as a cancer agent. The list of carcinogens now linked with specific occupations, food additives, and environmental contaminants swells with almost unreal speed—like a horror movie monster —at first the size of an ordinary house fly, but suddenly huge enough to overwhelm whole cities.

In *Cancer Care*, written by two M.D.s, Drs. Harold Glucksburg and Jack W. Singer, the modern situation is summarized: "It has been estimated that up to 80 percent of all cancers are caused or influenced by carcinogens. Until recently, man lived and evolved in a relatively stable and natural environment. This is no longer true. Since the industrial revolution, a dazzling variety of new synthetic products, the effects of which are at best unknown, have been introduced into the environment. We have altered our environment more in the past decade than in the previous millennium."

Like the children's puzzle with pictures that seem intact at first glance but actually conceal several mistakes, such as an upsidedown door or a chimney poking out of the side of a house, our familiar surroundings and daily routines are perforated with cancerous flaws. Publicizing risks has become the daily routine of researchers and media. But bombarded with data, we begin to feel powerless, at times even paranoid.

Then we read of the macrobiotic case histories which indicate the recovery from degenerative disease and discover a possible strategy to overcome cancer. These stories point to hope in a desperate morass of confusion and unknowns.

Again and again, patients call to inquire as to why macrobiotics can heal, and for what reason does the more customary diet hinder health. Although a great deal is yet to be charted scientifically, ample information can be found in medical literature right now. Dr. Block has combed current and old issues of medical periodicals, analyzing data and synthesizing research reports, in order to present the following correlations between food and disorders.

In the foods we eat, additives and preservatives might not be the only culprits that lead to cancer. Some of the familiar staples on the American dinner table have been implicated. Specifically, animal products and refined carbohydrates, which still make up the bulk of the American diet, contain substances which seem to promote disease. Let us review each in more detail.

The Overconsumption of Saturated Fat and Protein

Excessive amounts of saturated fats and cholesterol are abundant in animal foods and dairy products, like beef and butter. Besides the connection between fats and heart/vascular disorders, there is world-wide evidence linking lipids with several forms of cancer. Take colon/rectal cancer for example, one of the most common cancers in the United States. According to a recent study done by Dr. J. P. Cruse and his associates at the University College Hospital Medical School in London, fat consumption has been spotlighted as a cause.

In studying population groups, the highest incidence of colon cancer is witnessed in countries with the highest meat consumption; for example, the United States, Canada, Scotland, and New Zealand. In Japan, where there is less fat intake, bowel cancer occurs less than one-third as frequently as in the U.S. However, if Japanese migrate to the States and adopt a modern, Western diet with its reliance on meat and dairy, they show the same colon cancer statistics as other Americans.*

Table 5   National Cancer Rates
(World Health Organization, 1973)

Cancer site	Death rate per 100,000 population	
	U.S.	Japan
Intestine (male)	17.2	4.6
(female)	19.3	5.0
Breast	29.6	5.4

* Please refer to the Appendix at the end of this Chapter for additional data.

A fat-laden diet is the chief suspect in other cancers as well. According to the National Cancer Institute, fats accelerate the growth of breast tumors. Hormonal imbalance produced by fats is one explanation given by the American Health Foundation's Dr. Ernst Wynder. In his research he has established that the pancreas, kidney and bladder are also victimized by high fat intake.

In our modern day protein panic, the average person in this country annually consumes 193 pounds of red meat, 53 pounds of poultry, 294 eggs, and 375 pounds of dairy products (including cheese and other milk products). We have been hooked on a protein-need myth, when actually we might be consuming more than four times the protein we require. The present tendency is to assume that "more is better."

The truth is—excessive animal protein intake can jeopardize our health. High protein causes high ammonia levels in the intestines. Dr. Willard Visek, professor of clinical sciences at the University of Illinois Medical School explains: "Ammonia behaves like chemicals that cause cancer or promote its growth. It kills cells . . . and it increases the mass of the lining of the intestines. What is intriguing is that within the colon the incidence of cancer parallels the concentration of ammonia."

Even more data exist. In a 1975 issue of the *Journal of Cancer Research*, a high protein diet has been linked to bladder cancer as well as intestinal malignancies. Hesitate before reaching for a second helping and consider this fact. Regardless of the food ingested, excess eating or just plain gorging and gulping can increase tumor size and occurrence.

Excessive Dairy Consumption

Many of us have the impression that milk is a pure and wholesome food. However, its fresh, white appearance can be deceiving. Even after processing, milk is still not free of contaminants. An investigation of the Consumers' Union, published in a January 1974 issue of *Consumer Reports*, discovered bacterial counts exceeding 130,000 per milliliter in 7 test samples, although government standards declare safe limits at a maximum of 20,000 bacteria per milliliter (about 1/5 teaspoon). In fact, one sample contained as much as 3,000,000, and a few contained numbers too large to measure accurately.

In addition, 21 out of 25 tested milk brands were contaminated with pesticides. Health officials concur that there is no level of pesticides in milk that can be judged safe. Also detected in 21 of the milks analyzed were residues of chlorinated hydrocarbons. As they accumulate in the body, these hydrocarbons are not only capable of producing genetic mutations that result in birth defects but also have the potential of forming malignancies.

Added to this is the possibility that the cow milked for the glass you are now filling or for the slice of cheese on your plate might have been infected with bovine C-type virus. In laboratory experiments, this virus produced leukemia in test animals.

More and more, as explained by Frank Oski, M.D. in his book *Don't Drink*

Your Milk, we begin to realize that milk and milk products might not be the benign foods we think they are. Somewhere between eighteen months and four years, most people begin to lose lactase activity, an enzyme action in the intestines that breaks down lactase, the natural sugar present in milk. Since this decline in lactase is a normal process of maturing, perhaps it was never nature's intention for us to drink milk or eat foods with lactase after the weaning age.

In fact, the vast majority—over two-thirds of people on this earth—are lactase intolerant. So if you continue to drink milk, you might be setting yourself up for a myriad of problems. Some of these include overactivity of mucous secreting glands, infection, and possibly even malignant disease, according to William Crook, who explains the perils of allergenic foods in an article in *Pediatric Clinics of North America.*

Perhaps the most serious indictment of milk and foods derived from milk are the dangers of vitamin D excess and calcification from synthetic vitamin D. In separate medical papers, two M.D.s, Drs. M. Seelig and H. Taussig, have reported the dangerously high, actually toxic levels of vitamin D in our excess consumption of fortified milk products.

In 1953 the problem was aggravated. Major food processors found that it was less expensive to enrich products with an artificial form of the D vitamin, D_2, rather than fortifying with the true form, D_3. In extensive tests conducted by Dr. Hans Selye, a Nobel prize researcher, vitamin D_2 was linked with "Calciphylaxis" or calcium plaquing. There is ample evidence that many diseases, from arteriosclerosis to kidney stones, can be traced to this deleterious process of calcification. Microscopic examinations of cancer tumors frequently reveal calcium deposits. Why this link between tumors and calcification occurs, science has not yet documented. But the fact remains, the connection does exist.

Refined Carbohydrates and Sugar

Refined carbohydrates and processed foods have been judged guilty of many modern day woes. One of the most obvious is tooth decay. But the hazards of sugar are considerable. It plays an active role in such disorders as hyperactivity and diabetes, and creates susceptibility to polio, other infectious diseases, ulcers, and heart disease. Add to this catalogue of incriminations—cancer.

In a study commissioned by Hoffman-La Roche, Inc., sucrose (sugar) and xylitol (a substance used to sweeten sugarless gum) were found to produce malignant liver tumors. Although the test results were released in March 1978, the FDA did not discuss them with the Federal Trade Commission until the following year. Many researchers believe that if sugar were first introduced today, it would stand little chance of being approved by the FDA for mass consumption. Due to these laboratory tests, xylitol is not used commonly today, while sugar is still ever-present. In fact, it is almost impossible to wander through the grocery aisles and locate a can or package that does not include sugar in its contents. Moreover, sugar can be cleverly concealed on labels behind an alias like "sucrose" or "dextrose."

Solution: 1—Whole Cereal Grains

In travelling from farm field to grocery shelf, processed and packaged grain products have been stripped of most vitamins and minerals. Robbed of nature's rich nutrients, these refined carbohydrates are then stuffed with artificial supplements. In contrast, whole grains are "the real thing."

Professor Paul C. Mangelsdorf in the July 1963 issue of *Scientific American* made this definitive statement: "Cereal grains . . . represent a five-in-one food supply which contains carbohydrates, proteins, fats, minerals, and vitamins. A whole grain cereal, if its food values are not destroyed by the over-refinement of modern processing methods, comes closer than any other plant product to providing an adequate diet."

Whole grains heal the body as well as fuel it. High fiber, the stuff of cereal grains, reduces the risk of colon and other cancers. As an additional bonus, grains produce a beneficial form of cholesterol. Unlike the harmful type associated with animal foods, this favorable cholesterol actually breaks down dangerous saturated fat and oil residue.

Perhaps most impressive is the role grains can play in strengthening the entire immunologic system, the body's equipment in combatting disease. A May 1980 issue of *Hosptial Tribune* reports that diseases stemming from a weak immune system "are associated with a high incidence of malignancies."

Three vitamins in particular are essential to immunity: pyridoxine (vitamin B_6), folic acid, and pantothenic acid. All are plentiful in whole grains. According to Dr. A. E. Axelrod of Pittsburgh University Medical School, if any one of these three is absent from the diet, the body cannot manufacture antibodies (proteins that fight disease). Unfortunately, it is these three elements of the B-complex that are left on the milling room floor in the refining process. Therefore, they are not present in white bread, white flour products, white rice, or even degerminated cornmeal. The implications of this are tremendous: A natural, whole grain diet can build resistance to disease, while a refined foods diet does not.

Solution: 2—*Miso*

Philippe Shubik said in *Potential Carcinogenicity of Food Additives and Contaminants*, "Since it might not be possible to remove all carcinogenic materials from the environment, methods to mitigate or neutralize their harmful effects should be sought." Surprisingly, the sought-after substance might not emerge from chemical laboratories and test-tube concoctions but from less obvious sources: fermented soybeans and sea vegetables.

Miso (pronounced mee-so), a deep and rich tasting fermented soybean purée, appears regularly in macrobiotic menus, especially soups and condiments. An excellent provider of protein, B_{12} and other nutrients, it boasts properties that work almost like magic in the body. When the atomic bomb was dropped on Nagasaki in 1945, Dr. Akizuki, director of Urakami Hospital, made certain that his entire staff was fed *miso* soup daily. Exposure to radiation was unavoidable;

his hospital was located only one mile from the center of the blast. In follow-up studies, he discovered that none of his co-workers suffered from the devastating effects of atomic radiation. Other comparable groups were not as fortunate. He hypothesized that *miso* was the protective factor.

Almost thirty years later, in 1972, Japanese scientists who were stimulated by Dr. Akizuki's records identified *Zybicolin* in *miso*. This substance, a byproduct of the *natto* and *miso* yeasts, has been found to collect and then remove from the body heavy molecules—metals, pollutants, and radioactive poisons.

Miso has a repertoire of other benefits. For one, it is richly endowed with lecithin and linoleic acid. Each of these dissolves, then eliminates cancer-linked cholesterol and fat accumulations. Another benefit: An acid blood condition is like a door thrust open to disease. *Miso* helps to shut this door by modulating an acid blood level into a healthy alkaline level. And an additional bonus: Present in all nonpasteurized *miso* are active enzymes, particularly *lactobacillus*, which aid the digestive flora.

Solution: 3—Sea Vegetables

If someone mentions treasures from the sea, we usually picture pirate chests bursting with gold pieces. Actually, simple plants growing in the ocean yield rich bounties for our health and well-being.

Put aside your vitamin capsules and mineral supplements. Sea grown vegetables furnish copious amounts of vitamins A, B, and C. One variety *kombu*, a popular macrobiotic soup ingredient, has three times more B vitamins than milk or milk products. And ergosterol, which converts to vitamin D (the natural version, D_3) in the body, is richly supplied by all sea plants.

In addition, mineral assets are high in sea vegetables. For example, an average portion of *hijiki* provides fourteen times the quantity of calcium found in a glass of milk. No other food source can claim as great a concentration of iron as dulse. Another boon: Research has found that cancer sufferers excrete vital amounts of zinc; kelp readily replenishes this essential element.

Besides this rich inventory of vitamins, minerals and basic nutrients, sea vegetables, actually inhibit the absorption of radioactive strontium and cadmium. Further, in research at McGill University, Montreal, alginates demonstrated the ability to bind with heavy, toxic molecules within the intestines and then to change them into insoluble salts which are finally excreted from the body.

Unlike prescription medications, whole grains, *miso* and sea vegetables do not produce the harmful side effects often connected with drugs. Macrobiotics is, therefore, not only good food. It is also good medicine.

Summary

It is sad truth that in the declared "war against cancer" no new drug treatment nor modern medical technology has produced any true victories. According to Dr. Robert Mendelsohn, author of *Confessions of a Medical Heretic* and former chairman of the Medical Licensing Board of the State of Illinois, "In the closing decades of the twentieth century, the great scourges of our time are heart disease and cancer; both are regarded as mysterious and despite (or because of?) all the efforts of modern medicine, still incurable." Thus, macrobiotics is not only good medicine, it might be one of the few effective ones.

However, some patients discover that switching from American staples to a macrobiotic diet might not be a simple one-step procedure. For many people, changing the foods they eat means changing their lives. Realigning personal priorities is involved. Each of us must weigh the importance of our health against the comfort of our habits.

Perhaps cancer will not become an obsolete term in this, or even the next generation. But shrugging our shoulders in despair and surrendering to disease are not necessary. Even though we cannot immediately purge all the carcinogens from our external environment, we can, as promptly as our next meal, begin to clean house internally.

Today we are suffering from an epidemic of degenerative disease. The appalling statistics tell the story: one out of five Americans developing diabetes at some point in their lifetime; one out of four with arthritis; one out of three with cardio-vascular disease; and, by the year 2000, if our decay continues unabated, many of us believe cancer will hit every other individual.

We in the macrobiotic community around the world believe that this is com-pletely unnecessary. The way to change our present state of health is not through political, economic, or psychological measures, but through biological ones. For our communities to become well again, each of us must examine our personal way of life and most importantly, our dietary habits.

The answer to our problems will not be found through further technological advancement. As a physician, it is my hope that the 1980s will bring about a more conservative approach to medicine, one in which the excessive use of high tech-nology and drugs is deemed counterproductive both from the economic and biological standpoints.

In the years ahead, each of us must return to the underlying cause of our society's and our own personal condition. Once determined, it will become very clear that through proper dietary practices and a return to more traditional living patterns, we can remedy our present situation. The macrobiotic way of life and its age old system of health care can address these needs.

Data on the Relationship between Diet and Cancer

Much of the scientific data linking cancer and diet has come from two sources: (1) *epidemiological data*, such as that which correlates the incidence of various types of cancer with dietary patterns in the United States, Japan, and other countries, and (2) *animal studies*, such as those which suggest that a restriction of caloric or protein intake may have an inhibiting effect on the development of cancer. Examples of both varieties of data are presented below. Several of these examples were initially compiled in the 1977 *Status Report* of the Diet, Nutrition, and Cancer Program of the National Cancer Institute.

Epidemiological Data

1. *The decline in cancer incidence in Holland following World War II food shortages.* Between 1942 and 1946, the incidence of cancer in Holland dropped 35 to 60 percent, depending on the area of the country. A Dutch epidemiologist, Dr. F. de Waard, has correlated this decline with the changes in diet which occurred as a result of the German occupation of the country. During the occupation, the Germans requisitioned most of the cheese, butter, milk, eggs, and meat in the country, forcing the Dutch to live on home-grown vegetables, bread, and other basic staples. With the return of normal conditions after the war, the cancer rates jumped back to their pre-war levels.

2. *Changes in cancer incidence among Japanese migrants to the United States following the adoption of a high-fat and high-protein diet.* As discussed in Chapter 1 the rates of colon and breast cancer in Japan are relatively low, while stomach cancer is high. The opposite is true in the United States. Within three generations, however, Japanese immigrants in this country shift from the cancer incidence patterns common in Japan to those common in the United States. This shift correlates with a change from the standard Japanese way of eating to the modern American one, with a corresponding increase in the intake of calories, fat, and protein. A nutritional comparison between the average Japanese and American diet is presented in Table 6.

Table 6   **Nutrition in the U.S. and Japan**
(Hirayama, 1975)

Nutrient	U.S.	Japan	Percent of U.S. value
Food energy (cal.)	3300	2273	69
Protein (g)	99	84	85
Fat (g)	155	52	34
Carbohydrate (g)	385	351	91
Calcium (g)	0.95	0.55	58
Vitamin A (IU)	8100	2043	25
Riboflavin (mg)	2.32	0.98	42

Fig. 16 Large Bowel Cancer Mortality and Dietary Fat and Oil Consumption
(Wynder, 1975)

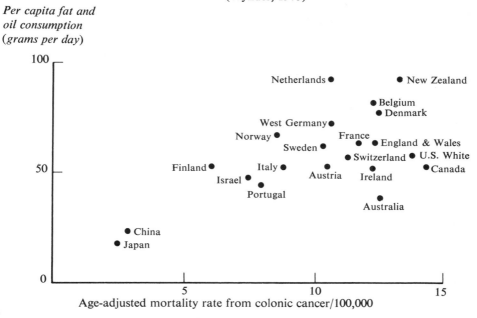

Per capita fat and oil consumption (grams per day)

Age-adjusted mortality rate from colonic cancer/100,000

Fig. 17 Relationship between Breast Cancer and Dietary Fat Intake
(Carroll, 1975)

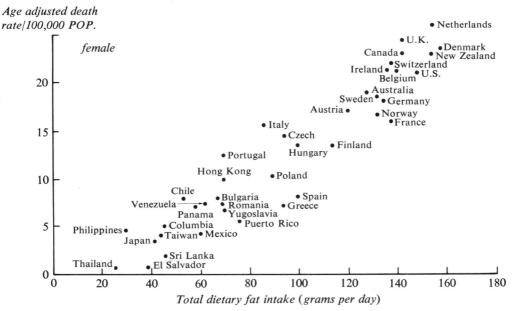

Age adjusted death rate/100,000 POP.

Total dietary fat intake (grams per day)

3. The worldwide correlation between a high meat and fat intake and a high incidence of breast and colon cancer. In countries where the intake of meat and animal fat is high, such as Scotland, Canada, and the United States, the mortality rates from colonic and breast cancer are also high. Countries such as Japan and Chile, where meat consumption is low, have a correspondingly low incidence of these diseases. (See Figs. 16 and 17.)

The difference between the high incidence of these illnesses in the United States and their low incidence in Japan is consistent with the differences in fat intake between the two countries, and correlates with the increase in the incidence of colon cancer in Japanese migrants to the U.S. following their adoption of Western dietary habits.

Evidence from specific population groups within the United States also reinforces this connection. Groups such as the Seventh-Day Adventists, who generally follow a semi-vegetarian regime with a limited fat and meat intake, have a much lower rate of some forms of cancer, especially breast and colon. These diseases have also been found to correlate with a low intake of cereal grains which contain dietary fiber. For example, certain African populations who, like the Japanese, have a low-fat, light-fiber regimen, have been found to have correspondingly low incidences of colon cancer. The same appears true for the Seventh-Day Adventists.

4. The increasing incidence of breast and colon cancer in Japan following Westernization of the Japanese diet. The rising consumption of milk and milk products, meat, eggs, oil, and fat which has occurred in Japan since World War II (see Fig. 18) correlates with an increase in the incidences of breast and colon cancer over the last twelve years. According to the National Cancer Institute, this increase is "consistent with the Westernization of the Japanese diet during recent decades, particularly with an increased intake of fat."

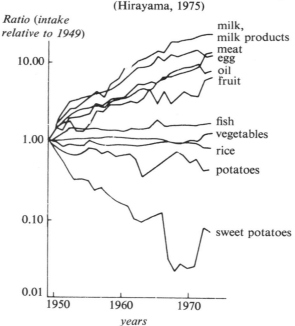

Fig. 18   Change in Intake of Selected Foods in Japan
(Hirayama, 1975)

5. Evidence indicating that the inclusion of fresh vegetables in the daily diet may protect against lung cancer. A recently completed nineteen-year study of 3,100 Chicago area men conducted by Dr. Mark Lepper of Rush-Presbyterian-St. Luke's Medical Center and Dr. Oglesby Paul of Harvard Medical School, seems to indicate that a diet which includes daily servings of dark leafy greens, carrots, squash, and other vegetables helps protect against lung cancer. In this study, men who ate regular servings of these vegetables had up to eight times less risk of lung cancer than those who ate infrequent servings. The study found that the protective effect of these vegetables increased with the quantity eaten.

Animal Studies

1. Studies which show that a restriction of calories inhibits the development of tumors. A number of animal studies have shown that of all dietary modifications tried so far, the restriction of food intake has had the most regular influence on the development of tumors. A restriction in overall caloric intake has been regularly found to inhibit the formation of tumors and increase life expectancy of experimental animals. Similar trials have also shown that among rats fed identical diets, the incidence of tumors is consistently higher in heavier animals.

2. Studies which reveal a higher incidence of tumors in animals which are fed high-protein diets. According to the NCI report, a lower protein intake inhibits the development of spontaneous or chemically induced tumors. Comparison of 5 percent and 20 percent casein diet on aflatoxin induced tumors showed rats on the higher protein diet had 50 percent greater incidence of cancer. All of the high protein rats developed tumors or precancerous lesions, while those on the lower protein diet had no tumors or precancerous lesions.

3. Studies which show a relationship between a high-fat diet and a higher incidence of breast and colon cancer. A number of studies have shown that an increase in the amount of fat in animal diets produces an increase in the incidence of certain cancers, and that the cancers tend to develop earlier in the life of the animal. According to the NCI report, "Tannenbaum has shown that an increase from 25 to 28 percent fat in the diet of mice resulted in a double incidence of spontaneous mammary cancers."

4. Studies which suggest that a natural food diet contains "protective factors" for the prevention of cancer. In one group of studies quoted in the NCI report, irridated mice consuming a natural foods diet had a markedly lower incidence of tumors than similar mice receiving a highly refined diet. According to the report, these studies suggest "the presence of a protective factor in natural food diets."

A Summary of the Evidence

In June, 1982, a report entitled, *Diet, Nutrition, and Cancer* was issued by an expert panel of the National Academy of Sciences. After reviewing the accumulating evidence linking diet and cancer, the panel recommended the following dietary guidelines:

Cut consumption of foods high in saturated and unsaturated fats to 30 percent of daily calories. The panel suggested that consumption of both saturated and unsaturated fats be reduced by 25 percent, primarily by eating less fatty meats, high fat dairy products, and fats and oils used in cooking and at the table. High fat diets have been linked especially to cancers of the colon, breast, and prostate.

Eat whole cereal grains, vegetables, and fruits on a daily basis. The panel pointed out that vegetables such as dark leafy greens, and deep yellow vegetables are excellent sources of beta-carotene, a substance associated with a reduced risk of many cancers, including cancer of the lung, breast, bladder, and skin. Cabbage, carrots, winter squash, broccoli, cauliflower, and brussels sprouts were recommended for their content of beta-carotene and other cancer inhibiting substances.

Eat few salt-cured, salt-pickled and smoked foods, such as sausages, smoked fish and ham, bacon bologna, and frankfurters. These foods increase exposure to a variety of carcinogenic substances, including nitrosamines and polycyclic hydrocarbons. Most of these foods are high in fat, and populations consuming them in large quantities tend to develop many cancers of the digestive tract.

Drink alcohol in moderation.

The thirteen member scientific committee which drafted the recommendations stated that diet could be responsible for up to 40 percent of cancer in men and 60 percent in women. "Most common cancers are potentially perventable, for they appear to be determined more by habit, diet, and custom than by genetic differences," the panel concluded. Paul Van Nevel, a spokesman for the National Cancer Institute, which commissioned the study, said that the report involved no new research but was the most extensive study to date of the relationship of diet and nutrition to cancer. "It was an exhaustive survey of all the research and literature worldwide and involved scientists from a wide range of disciplines," he said. Dr. Clifford Grobstein, chairman of the panel and an experimental biologist at the University of California in San Diego, said, "the evidence is increasingly impressive that what we eat does affect our chances of getting cancer." He suggested that the advice be followed without delay, "given the long time frame over which most cancers develop." The panel stated that the evidence it reviewed "suggests that cancers of most major sites are influenced by dietary patterns."

The recommendations put forward by the panel are similiar to those issued by the Senate Select Committee on Nutrition and Human Needs in the 1977 report, *Dietary Goals for the United States*. For a discussion of how the Standard Macrobiotic Diet fulfills the Dietary Goals, please refer to *Diet, Heart Disease, and Macrobiotics* in the following chapter.

Chapter 3

Diet and Heart Disease

Lessons from the Framingham Heart Study

William P. Castelli, M.D.

We are all part of the great American epidemic of coronary heart disease (CHD). Why do people call what is going on an epidemic? Look at Fig. 19 and what happened to Americans living in Framingham in just the first fourteen years of our study. We took every other man and woman who lived in Framingham into our study and examined them every two years to see who got a heart attack.

Fig. 19 Framingham Study; Fourteen-year-incidence of Coronary Heart Disease (All Clinical Manifestations) in Men and Women Thirty to Sixty-two Years of Age at Entry into Study

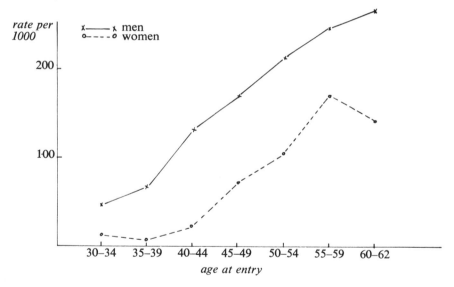

Fig. 20 shows what happened to 5,127 men and women. If you look at men aged forty to forty-four, every eighth man developed some form of coronary heart disease in that first year period. Every sixth man aged forty-five to forty-nine, every fifth man aged fifty to fifty-four, every fourth man fifty-five years or older developed CHD in just those first fourteen years. Women ran much lower rates prior to the menopause (age forty-five) and then started to catch up to the men. Of course, the worst statistic of all concerns what happened to people in Framingham younger on—prior to the age of sixty. By age sixty, every fifth man and every

Fig. 20 Diagramatic Representation of the Plasma Lipoprotein Subclasses and Their Separation Using Either Electrophoresis or Ultracentrifugal Sedimentation

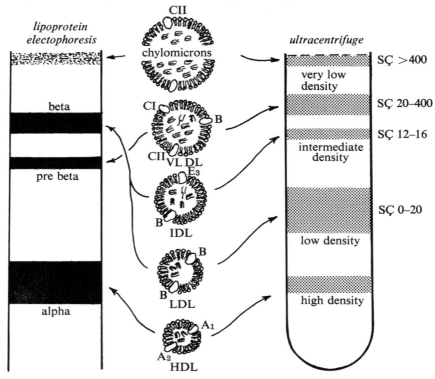

seventeenth woman in the town had developed some form of CHD. These people are still relatively young—they are in their forties and fifties.

The process which causes a heart attack is what we call atherosclerosis, and this leads to a disease of the heart called coronary heart disease. Atherosclerosis is simple; the deposition of fats, primarily a kind of cholesterol called cholesterol ester, in the linings of our blood vessels. Our blood vessels are like pipes carrying blood which has food and oxygen to our cells. Atherosclerosis blocks these pipes with fatty and tissue deposits which impede the flow of blood to the cells of our heart or brain or any other organ. The worst occurs when the process of atherosclerosis combines finally with a blood clot to completely shut down the blood flow. When that happens to our heart, a process called myocardial infarction, or death of part of our heart muscle, occurs. When it happens in the brain, a stroke occurs. When it happens in our legs we may have a leg amputated. The process of atherosclerosis is very complex, but one of the most essential ingredients in the process is to have too high a level of the blood fats, particularly the wrong kind of cholesterol.

Now the cholesterol in our diet is carried around in fat particles which we call the lipoproteins. These lipoproteins are depicted in Fig. 20. We actually know how all the different molecules are arranged in these particles and we understand how the body makes and disperses of most of them. All the particles carry cholesterol, so it is as if we all have five different kinds of cholesterol in our blood. Are all these cholesterols equally atherogenic? We feel the worst kind is LDL cholesterol. LDL stands for "low density lipoprotein" cholesterol, a form which is derived from the way we separate out these lipoproteins in an ultra centrifuge. In an ultra centrifuge these particles layer out according to size. IDL cholesterol, VLDL cholesterol, and chylomicron cholesterol are certainly not good for us when they become elevated in our blood, so these four cholesterols form the "gang of four" bad cholesterols. The other cholesterol in our blood is called HDL (high density lipoprotein) cholesterol, and the more we have the better we seem to do. The *Reader's Digest* (February, 1978) called HDL the "good cholesterol." How we turn out in life—whether we get a heart attack or not—depends on the balance of these cholesterols, the good and the bad in our bloodstream.

Diet is related in a very important way to the level of our blood cholesterols. Animal meats contain mostly cholesterol and saturated fat; two kinds of fat which elevate our bad cholesterols—particularly LDL cholesterol—which many feel is the major cholesterol deposited in our blood vessel walls. Polyunsaturated fat, which is found in vegetable oils like corn oil, safflower oil, sunflower seed oil, and others lowers the bad cholesterols in our blood. Egg yolks rich in cholesterol are to be avoided. Dairy fat is likewise dangerous, because it raises the bad cholesterols. Things that raise the good cholesterol HDL are fish, weight loss, exercise, onions, and vitamin E, which is naturally available in whole grains and vegetable oils. A vegetarian produces the best balance of HDL cholesterol to the bad cholesterols and is thus a very favorable undertaking in general. Some people say that because our body manufactures cholesterol it does not matter what we eat, but this is totally false. *People who eat little saturated fat or cholesterol have cholesterols so low in this country that they virtually appear to be immune to this disease.* When the body does not get very much saturated fat or cholesterol in the diet our cholesterols average about 125 mg. percent instead of the usual 225 mg. percent found in Framingham.

Some unfortunate people inherit a tendency to make one or more of the different cholesterols at an accelerated rate. (Depending on which type of particle is elevated we talk of type I, II, III, IV, or V.) The worst genetic tendency results in elevated levels of LDL cholesterol, called the type II hyperlipoproteinemia. These people are not rare; about one in twenty Americans has this tendency. People with this disorder develop CHD early in life, often by the age of forty. Another common disorder is the type IV; this is due to an elevation of the VLDL cholesterol particle where actually most of the triglyceride, another kind of fat in our blood, is carried. So not only do these people have too much cholesterol, but they have very high levels of triglyceride. Such genetically disposed people have to pay very strict attention to the foods they eat, because they convert most of the fat in an American diet into the wrong kind of cholesterol.

Very early on in the Framingham Heart Study, which has been going on for thirty-two years now, it was learned that the higher the level of LDL cholesterol or VLDL cholesterol, where 90 percent of the bad cholesterols are carried in our blood, the higher the subsequent rate of CHD. *It seems as though the rich diet of animal fats and dairy fats was converted to the bad cholesterols, which in turn were deposited in our blood vessels to produce atherosclerosis, or the clogging of these vessels by fat deposits.* About fourteen years ago we began to measure HDL cholesterols and found the higher these went in our blood the lower was the subsequent rate of CHD.

The HDL cholesterol story is an interesting one. Why should a cholesterol in our blood be good for us? What is it doing? The story that is currently unfolding suggests that HDL goes out to the deposits of cholesterol in our blood vessels and picks up the cholesterol there and initiates a process that brings it back to our liver where 95 percent of the cholesterol we excrete per day from our bodies is excreted through our bile ducts into our small intestines. The higher our HDL cholesterol, the lower is our total body cholesterol. It appears thus that the body has a mechanism for getting rid of cholesterol deposits. Is atherosclerosis reversible? Why not; the body has a biochemical pathway to undo the deposits of fat in our blood vessels.

One of the most important issues of the 1980's will be the question of reversibility of atherosclerosis in clinical medicine. Most doctors in this country have been taught that atherosclerosis is not reversible, but we now know that in most of the animal studies you can take animals with almost 90 percent of their blood vessels blocked by fatty deposits and scar tissue and if you lower their cholesterols (total cholesterols) to 150 or lower, 80 percent of the lesions will disappear in about four years. *We are now seeing case reports in humans where this same thing has occurred.* A doctor in Nashville, Tennessee sent me pictures of x-rays he had taken of a patient who had a 90 percent occlusion of one of the main arteries of his heart. Now usually such people get what is known as bypass surgery. That is to say a surgeon will take a vein from your leg and run it around the blockage in your heart's blood vessel. Indeed, this patient from Nashville had a bypass in 1973, but he went on a vegetarian diet. Five years later he came back to his doctor and told him how well he felt and that he felt so well he was sure he had reversed all the blockages in the blood vessel to his heart. Of course, the doctor thought he was crazy—even asked him what medical school he went to. However, because the patient was persistent, in order to shut the patient up, the doctor repeated the x-ray studies of the blood vessels of the patient's heart and to everyone's surprise, all the deposits of fat (atherosclerosis) had disappeared!

A vegetarian diet you say—I always thought the vegetarians were the "nuts among the berries." Well, we should look at these vegetarians. In a study of 18,000 vegetarians in California, Dr. Phillips of Loma Linda Unversity found that they only run about 15 percent of our heart attack rate. Not only that, they only run 40 percent of our cancer rate and perhaps best of all, their men live six to seven years longer than our men; their women live three years longer than our women. If vegetarians are so crazy, why are they doing so much better than us?

While the few case reports in humans showing reversibility are encouraging people; many wonder how universal might this process of reversibility be. One clue comes from the experience in Europe during the Second World War. Two years after the German occupation of Belgium, Holland, Poland, and Norway, virtually all the atherosclerosis or fatty deposits in the blood vessels had disappeared. Such deposits were present in 70 percent of the autopsies done before the war, but from 1942 to 1950 they disappeared. Now, after the war, 70 percent of the people get these deposits in their blood vessels as do 70 percent of the people in America. Where did these deposits go during World War II? Of course, these people were in semi-starvation. *We have seen in Framingham that no one whose cholesterols stayed below 150 mg. percent developed CHD in the first twenty-five years of our study.* This is similar to what we see in Asia, Africa, and South America, outside the big cities; namely that cholesterols are very low compared to America and that coronary heart disease is virtually unkown. We have, with Dr. Frank Sacks, studied over 200 macrobiotic vegetarians in the New England area and their average cholesterol was 125 to 150 mg. percent.[1]

I recently visited Japan where for years the Japanese have been spared the devastation of coronary heart disease, even though they smoked and had very high levels of blood pressure (from eating too much salt). Of course, this was largely thanks to their diet built around rice, fish, and vegetables. The fat intake in the Japanese diet was 40–50 grams per day, not 70–120 grams as we eat in America. Unfortunately, this is changing in Japan. Japanese economic success has allowed them to import more meat and cheese, which they are doing and in some studies in the Tokyo area, the fat content of their diet has almost reached 70 grams. Their heart attack rate is climbing at an alarming rate. This is a terrible proof of the cholesterol theory. One other point, in Japan and in Thailand I was very disappointed to see that brown rice is giving way to white rice in Asia. It is unfortunate to see that happen.

One final perspective. Our studies in Framingham suggest that the best way to learn how a person whose cholesterol is over 150 mg. percent will do is to determine the ratio of his or her total cholesterol to HDL cholesterol. For example, a man with a total cholesterol of 200 and an HDL of 50 would have a ratio of 200/50 or 4. We recommend that as a first practical step, Americans should try to get their ratio below 4.5. The reason for this is that the bulk of Americans who get a heart attack have a ratio of 4.6 to 5.7. While just getting one's total cholesterol to HDL cholesterol below 4.5 would not eliminate heart attack in this country, it would certainly remove heart attack as the number one killer in the U.S. Of course, if I say to all Americans, get your ratio below 4.5, I am telling half the women over thirty in this country to go on a diet; and about 60–70 percent of the men would have to do likewise. The macrobiotic vegetarians we studied, incidently, had a ratio of 2.5. Boston marathon runners were at 3.4. These are ratios at which we rarely, if ever, see coronary heart disease.

What a person puts into their mouths every day is a very important aspect of how they will do in life. More people need to take a critical look at how they are doing in that regard!

---

[1] Strictly speaking, these macrobiotic "vegetarians" did not eschew all animal products. For a more complete explanation of what the macrobiotic diet involves, refer to Chapter 1 and the following article.

Diet, Heart Disease, and Macrobiotics

Lawrence H. Kushi

Most people first view macrobiotics in terms of the diet, either because of its purported ability to treat degenerative illnesses, or as the next step in a gradually evolving life-style. Additionally, those who view macrobiotics with skepticism invariably point to the diet as the basis for their caution and criticism. This orientation naturally results in a need for a greater awareness of what the "macrobiotic" diet is, and what "macrobiotics" actually encompasses. The following paragraphs will address the former need in the context of the current American epidemic of coronary heart disease.

In February of 1977, the United States Senate Select Committee on Nutrition and Human Needs published a booklet called "Dietary Goals for the United States." The motivating force behind the publication of this booklet was the steadily increasing scientific evidence that the current American dietary pattern was—and is—a major reason that Americans develop and die from coronary heart disease, as well as other degenerative illnesses.

Meanwhile, persons living a macrobiotic life-style have, for many years, been following a general dietary pattern that presaged the suggestions put forth in the dietary goals. For educational purposes this dietary pattern has come to be called the "Standard Macrobiotic Diet" and is described in detail elsewhere in this book.

How does the Standard Macrobiotic Diet compare with either the current American diet as described in "Dietary Goals for the United States," or with the dietary goals themselves? To answer this question, it is necessary to translate the Standard Macrobiotic Diet into sources of calories, as the dietary goals themselves are presented. This translation and a graphic comparison with the current American Diet and the dietary goals is given in Fig. 21. The seven dietary goals, as revised in December of 1977, are outlined below, annotated to emphasize how the Standard Macrobiotic Diet contributes toward the realization of these goals:

1. *To avoid overweight, consume only as much energy (calories) as is expended; if overweight, decrease energy intake and increase energy expenditure.* Casual observation of people who eat in accordance with macrobiotic dietary principles indicates a very low prevalence of obesity.
2. *Increase the consumption of complex carbohydrates and "naturally occurring" sugars from about 28 percent of energy intake to about 48 percent of energy intake.* With cereal grains supplemented by legumes and vegetables forming the staple of the Standard Macrobiotic Diet, the intake of complex carbohydrate is easily increased to over 70 percent of energy intake.
3. *Reduce the consumption of refined and processed sugars by about 45 percent to account for about 10 percent of energy intake.* Since the Standard Macrobiotic Diet emphasizes natural and minimally processed foods, refined and

Fig. 21 A Nutritional Comparison between the Current American Diet, the U.S. Dietary Goals, and the Standard Macrobiotic Diet

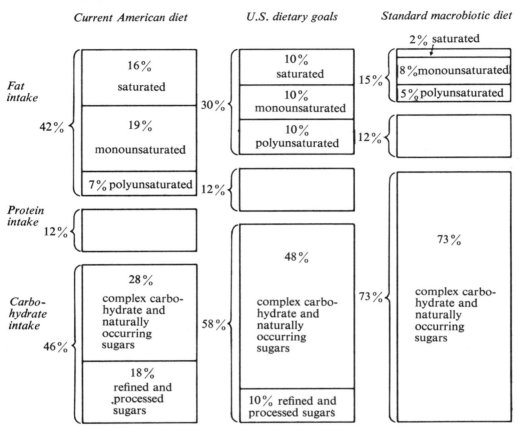

processed sugars form a negligible proportion of the energy intake of the diet.

4. *Reduce overall fat consumption from approximately 40 percent to about 30 percent of energy intake.* A very large proportion of the fat intake in the American diet comes from meat and dairy food, as well as through the processing of other foods. As these types of foods are generally not consumed in the Standard Macrobiotic Diet, fat consumption is reduced to about 15 percent of energy intake.

5. *Reduce saturated fat consumption to about 10 percent of total energy intake and balance that with polyunsaturated and monosaturated fats, which should account for about 10 percent of energy each.* The idea behind this goal is that, within a given amount of fat intake, one should attempt to balance the amount of saturated and polyunsaturated fat, such that polyunsaturated fats are consumed in equal or greater amounts than saturated fats. Since the major sources of fat in the Standard Macrobiotic Diet are oils existing in whole grains, legumes, and vegetables, or the liquid vegetables used for stir-frying, it is very difficult to consume more saturated fat than polyunsaturated fat. The best sources of saturated fat generally are animal foods,

hydrogenated fats, and coconut oil, while the best sources of polyunsaturated fats are liquid vegetable oils or whole grains.

6. *Reduce cholesterol consumption to about 300 milligrams a day.* Foods of animal origin are virtually the only source of cholesterol in the diet. Since the consumption of animal foods is de-emphasized in the Standard Macrobiotic Diet, only a nominal (much less than 300 mg.) amount of cholesterol is usually consumed.

7. *Limit the intake of sodium by reducing the intake of salt to about 5 grams a day.* A large proportion of sodium in the American diet comes from the intake of processed foods. Since foods in the Standard Macrobiotic Diet are at most only minimally processed, this is not a major source of sodium. However, the daily use of such foods as sea vegetables, *miso*, and *shoyu* add considerable amounts of sodium to the macrobiotic diet. The range of sodium intake on a macrobiotic diet has yet to be adequately quantified, but it is probably greater than 5 grams a day.

With the possible exception of Goal No. 7, the Standard Macrobiotic Diet surpasses the dietary goals. This is important to note, since the general consensus among nutrition professionals is that, in order to effectively impact on the health of the American population, a shift in dietary patterns in the same direction as, but more dramatic than, those set forth in the dietary goals is necessary. Note that the major sources of controversy that arose when "Dietary Goals for the United States" was published spoke to economic issues surrounding a dietary shift as proposed in the goals, rather than to health issues.

Although the actual mechanism by which diet leads to the development of heart disease is not totally clear, there are a number of plausible and probable ways in which this may occur. The dietary goals attempts to address many of these hypotheses, while the macrobiotic diet practically embraces most of them.

The best understood role of diet in the development of heart disease involves the role of fat and cholesterol in the diet. It is a virtual certainty that the consumption of too much fat, too much cholesterol, and too much saturated fat all influence the development of heart disease unfavorably. This is detailed in the preceding article by Dr. William Castelli. In contrast, the consumption of adequate amounts of complex carbohydrates and fiber may help prevent heart disease. Another hypothesis points to the possible role of animal protein in helping to advance the development of heart disease. And, it is probable that eating too much in general may also lead to heart disease. The more likely of these hypotheses is presented in Fig. 22.

We can anticipate the impact on heart disease that a shift in dietary patterns toward the Standard Macrobiotic Diet may have by looking at the risk factors of persons eating macrobiotically compared with persons eating the American diet. These risk factors, as shown by the Framingham study and other similar studies, include blood cholesterol levels, blood pressure, and cigarette smoking. That is, the higher the amount of cholesterol in the blood, the higher the blood pressure level, or the more cigarettes smoked, the greater the chance of eventually devel-

Fig. 22 How Diet May Influence Risk of Heart Disease

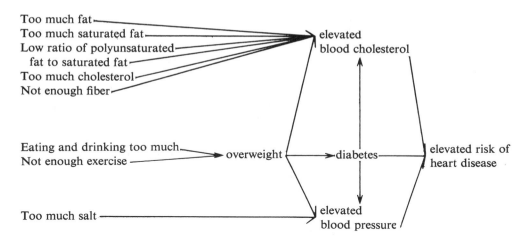

oping and dying from coronary heart disease. In addition, it is now clear that the amounts of the different types of cholesterol in the blood is important in determining the risk of heart disease. Thus, the relative amounts of the total cholesterol in the blood to the HDL (high density lipoprotein) cholesterol reflects risk of heart disease better than total blood cholesterol alone. The greater this ratio of total cholesterol to HDL cholesterol, the greater is the risk of heart disease.

Several studies have looked at the cholesterol or blood pressure levels among people eating macrobiotically. The first of these, published in 1974,[2] looked at the blood pressures of macrobiotic people living in the Boston area. It was found that these people had surprisingly low blood pressures, much lower than would have been expected. Was this due to eating little salt, or living a meditative unstressful life? It was apparent that salt intake was an unlikely explanation; in fact, of all the different variables looked at, only the amount of animal food consumed by these people consistently discriminated between those with higher and those with lower blood pressures.

Another observation about the blood pressure of these macrobiotic people gave credence to the idea that something environmental, such as the diet, was strongly influencing blood pressure levels. Previous studies of blood pressure showed that blood pressure levels tend to be similar within members of the same family, particularly if they live together. This "aggregation" of blood pressures has usually been attributed in part to genetic influences. Interestingly, this clustering was observed among the macrobiotic people only it did not occur within families. Many of the study participants lived in communal households, sharing the same food and to varying degrees having similar life-styles. It was within these households that the aggregation of blood pressures was observed. At least one of the interpretations given to this observation was that people who eat the same food tend to have similar blood pressures.

---

[2] Sacks, 1974.

The low blood pressures observed for macrobiotic people led to an investigation of both blood cholesterol and blood pressure among macrobiotic people, comparing them to a control population of persons living in Framingham of similar age and sex.[3] Once again, the blood pressures were much lower than expected, being much lower than the control population. It was expected that blood cholesterol levels would be lower in the macrobiotic population than in the Framingham population. Ample evidence from studies on people in metabolic wards who had their diets manipulated showed that blood cholesterol levels are influenced by diet, particularly by the amount of cholesterol in the diet.

The Boston-area macrobiotic people were indeed found to have much lower blood cholesterol levels than the non-macrobiotic people. Once again, however, the magnitude of the difference was surprising, as were the extremely low blood cholesterol levels. In fact, the cholesterol levels were among the lowest found in any human population anywhere in the world. In addition to the finding of extremely low blood cholesterol levels, the ratio of the amount of total cholesterol to the HDL cholesterol was found to be much lower for macrobiotic people, showing that this macrobiotic population was at negligible risk of developing heart disease.

The observation of extremely low total blood cholesterol levels in macrobiotic people has been confirmed in at least four other published studies, most recently in a study of macrobiotic people in Belgium and the Netherlands.[4] In Europe, as in Boston, macrobiotic people had cholesterol levels lower than other people, whether they were lacto-vegetarians or omnivores. The ratio of total cholesterol to HDL cholesterol was again found to be extremely favorable in terms of risk from heart disease.

A more controlled attempt to see if the macrobiotic diet per se was responsible for the extremely low blood pressures and cholesterol levels was the next logical step. Because of the possible role of animal food in determining blood pressure levels, a controlled study consisting of feeding portions of beef to people on a macrobiotic diet was carried out.[5] After eating their usual macrobiotic diet for a short period, these people then supplemented their diets with a portion of beef for one month. After this period, they returned to their usual diet without the beef.

As hypothesized, the blood pressures and cholesterol levels rose during the beef supplemented period, falling back to the low levels typical of macrobiotic people after the beef was removed from the diet. It was clear that the rise in cholesterol was due to the extra fat and cholesterol eaten as part of the beef, since the rise in cholesterol was of the magnitude that would have been predicted from previous studies in other groups. However, the rise in blood pressure was not as large as might have been expected from the large differences between macrobiotic people and omnivorous Americans. Further attempts to clarify the role of the macrobiotic diet in determining blood pressures are currently being conducted, focusing

---

[3] Sacks, 1975.
[4] Knuiman & West, 1982.
[5] Sacks, 1981.

on foods that are either not commonly eaten on a macrobiotic diet, or on foods that are almost unique to a macrobiotic diet.

It seems clear that the macrobiotic diet or one similar to it is the optimal diet in terms of reducing the risk of heart disease. What remains unclear is the magnitude of effect a change in diet will ultimately have on the prevention of heart disease.

The role of the macrobiotic diet in the prevention of heart disease will best be assessed by following the macrobiotic population over several years or decades to see what types of diseases develop in this group. But, based upon the known fact that macrobiotic people have extremely low blood pressures and cholesterol levels (summarized in Tables 7 and 8), and on the fact that vegetarian Seventh-Day Adventists have only fifteen percent of the rate of death from heart disease com-

Table 7   Blood Pressures in Macrobiotic People

Reference	Number of people	Systolic blood pressure (mm Hg)	Diastolic blood pressure (mm Hg)
Sacks, et al. (1974)			
men	127	109.7±11.5*	60.9±10.8
women	83	100.9± 9.3	58.2±12.0
Sacks, et al. (1975)			
macrobiotic	115	108.0±12.0	63.0±10.0
non-vegetarian	115	119.0±11.0	77.0± 8.0
Sacks, et al. (1981)	21	104.0	60.3

*Values are mean ± standard deviation.

Table 8   Cholesterol Levels of Macrobiotic People

Reference	Number of people	Total cholesterol (mg/dl)	HDL cholesterol (mg/dl)	Total/ HDL
Sacks, et al. (1975)				
macrobiotic	115	126±30*	43±11	2.9
non-vegetarian	115	184±37	49±12	3.8
Bergan & Brown (1980)				
men	44	148±32		
women	32	154±30		
East West Journal (1980)	11	121 (range: 102–147)		
Sacks, et al. (1981)	21	140	31**	4.5**
Knuiman & West (1982)				
men				
macrobiotic	33	146±35	46±12	3.2
non-vegetarian	52	212±39	46±12	4.3
boys				
macrobiotic	6	131±20	46±12	2.86
non-vegetarian	54	162±20	54±12	2.94

  * Values are mean ± standard deviation.
 ** Since the HDL cholesterol in this study was measured in blood specimens which had been frozen for three-and-a-half years, there was probably some deterioration of the HDL cholesterol. These figures are therefore unreliable.

pared with the general California population, it is probable that very few people eating macrobiotically will develop and die from heart disease.

Anecdotal evidence indicates that a change in dietary patterns from an American-style diet toward a macrobiotic diet will favorably enhance the survival of persons who have been diagnosed with coronary heart disease. This evidence is reinforced by the fact that reversibility of clinical heart disease has been observed in animals. What is needed to show the efficacy of the macrobiotic diet in the treatment of heart disease is a controlled clinical trial in which patients with heart disease are placed on a macrobiotic diet, and followed for a few years to determine how the diet influences their survival. Such a study is currently being planned by investigators at Harvard Medical School and one of the Harvard-affiliated hospitals. If this clinical trial turns out as is hoped, with patients put on a macrobiotic diet having much more favorable follow-ups than patients not on a macrobiotic diet, a major impact may be felt, changing the mode of treatment of heart disease.

The overall message seems clear. The risk of heart disease can be dramatically lowered by altering one's dietary pattern to one that conforms with the Standard Macrobiotic Diet. Even though the exact mechanisms by which this dietary shift influences this risk are unclear, it is known that such a shift does lead to risk reduction. Only the inertia behind the statement that heart disease is a multifactorial disease and therefore the effect of dietary change is unknown prevents dietary recommendations along the lines of the Standard Macrobiotic Diet from becoming a standard practice for the prevention of heart disease.

Excerpts from *Dietary Goals for the United States*

Introduction to the Second Edition

During this century, the composition of the average diet in the United States has changed radically. Foods containing complex carbohydrates and "naturally occurring"[6] sugars—fruit, vegetables and grain products—which were the mainstay of the diet, now play a minority role. At the same time, the consumption of fats and refined and processed sugars has risen to the point where these two macro-nutrients alone now comprise at least 60 percent of total caloric intake, an increase of 20 percent since the early 1900s.[7]

In the view of doctors and nutritionists consulted by the Select Committee, these and other changes in the diet amount to a wave of malnutrition—of both over- and under-consumption—that may be as profoundly damaging to the Nation's health as the widespread contagious diseases of the early part of the century.

The over-consumption of foods high in fat, generally, and saturated fat in particular, as well as cholesterol, refined and processed sugars, salt and/or alcohol has been associated with the development of one or more of six to ten leading causes of death: heart disease, some cancers, stroke and hypertension, diabetes, arteriosclerosis and cirrhosis of the liver. The associations are discussed more fully later in this report.

In his testimony at the Select Committee's July 1976 hearings on the relationship of diet to disease, Dr. Mark Hegsted of the Harvard School of Public Health, said:

> I wish to stress that there is a great deal of evidence and it continues to accumulate, which strongly implicates and, in some instances, proves that the major causes of death and disability in the United States are related to the diet we eat. I include coronary artery disease which accounts for nearly half of the deaths in the United States, several of the most important forms of cancer, hypertension, diabetes and obesity as well as other chronic diseases.

The over-consumption of food in general, combined with our more sedentary life-style, has become a major public health problem. In testimony at the same

---

[6] "Naturally occurring": Sugars which are indigenous to a food, as opposed to refined (cane and beet) and processed (corn sugar, syrups, molasses and honey) sugars which may be added to a food product.

[7] The food supply estimates are based on United States Department of Agriculture data showing the amounts of food that "disappear" into civilian channels.

hearings, Dr. Theodore Cooper, Assistant Secretary for Health, estimated that about 20 percent of all adults in the United States "are overweight to a degree that may interfere with optimal health and longevity."

At the same time, current dietary trends may also be leading to malnutrition through undernourishment. Fats are relatively low in vitamins and minerals, and refined sugar (cane and beet) and most processed sugars, have no vitamins and minerals. Consequently, diets with reduced caloric intake to control weight and/or save money, but which are high in fats and refined and processed sugars, may lead to vitamin and mineral deficiencies. As will be discussed later, low-income people may be particularly susceptible to inducements to consume diets high in fats, and refined and processed sugars.

The Department of Health, Education, and Welfare reported that health care expenditures in the United States in Fiscal Year 1976 totaled about $139.4 billion and predicted the cost could exceed $230 billion by Fiscal Year 1980. In testimony before the Select Committee in 1972, Dr. George Briggs, professor of nutrition at the University of California, Berkeley, estimated, based on a study by the Department of Agriculture, that improved nutrition might cut the Nation's health bill by one-third.

More recently, in an October 1977 letter to the Select Committee, Dr. Briggs provided an analysis of the cost of poor nutritional status which contributes to some of the diseases in the United States. The potential annual savings in nutrition related costs, "based on the more conservative end of the ranges of current scientific opinion," were as follows:

	(billion)
Dental diseases	$3
Diabetes	4
Cardiovascular disease	10
Alcohol	20
Digestive diseases	3
Total	$40

It should be noted that this analysis does not include cancer, kidney disease due to mismanagement of hypertension, or the long-term costs associated with low birthweight babies due to maternal malnutrition.

Beyond the monetary savings, it is obvious then that improved nutrition also offers the potential for prevention of vast suffering and loss of productivity and creativity.

One in three men in the United States can be expected to die of heart disease or stroke before age sixty and one in six women. It is estimated that 25 million suffer from high blood pressure and that about 5 million are afflicted by diabetes mellitus.[8]

---

[8] Statistics from reports and testimony presented to the Select Committee's National Nutrition ▶

Given the wide impact on health that has been traced to the dietary trends outlined, it is imperative, as a matter of public health policy, that consumers be provided with dietary guidelines or goals for macro-nutrients that will encourage the most healthful selection of foods.

Based on (1) testimony presented to the Select Committee in the ten days of hearings entitled "Diet Related to Killer Diseases" which began in July 1976 and ended in October 1977; (2) the Select Committee's 1974 National Nutrition Policy hearings; (3) guidelines established by governmental and professional bodies in the United States and at least eight other nations; and (4) a variety of expert opinion, the following Dietary Goals are recommended for the United States. Although genetic and other individual differences among health individuals exist, there is substantial evidence indicating that following these guidelines may be generally beneficial. (See preceding article for a discussion of the goals.)

Statements

Dr. D.M. Hegsted, former Professor of Nutrition, Harvard School of Public Health, Boston

The diet of the American people has become increasingly rich—rich in meat, other sources of saturated fat and cholesterol, and in sugar. There will be people who will contest this statement. It has been pointed out repeatedly that total sugar use has remained relatively constant for a number of years. We would emphasize, however, that our total food consumption has fallen even though we still eat too much relative to our needs. Thus, the proportion of the total diet contributed by fatty and cholesterol-rich foods and by refined foods has risen. We might be better able to tolerate this diet if we were much more active physically, but we are a sedentary people.

It should be emphasized that this diet which affluent people generally consume is everywhere associated with a similar disease pattern—high rates of ischemic heart disease, certain forms of cancer, diabetes, and obesity. These are the major causes of death and disability in the United States. These so-called degenerative diseases obviously become more important now that infectious diseases are, relatively speaking, under good control. I wish to emphasize that these diseases undoubtedly have a complex etiology. It is not correct, strictly speaking, to say that they are caused by malnutrition but rather that an inappropriate diet contributes to their causation. Our genetic makeup contributes—not all people are equally susceptible. Yet those who are genetically susceptible, most of us, are those who would profit most from an appropriate diet. Diet is one of the things that we can change if we want to.

▶ Policy hearings, June 1974, appearing in National Nutrition Policy Study, 1974, Part 6. June 21, 1974, heart disease, p. 2633; high blood pressure, p. 2529; diabetes, p. 2623.

There will undoubtedly be many people who will say we have not proven our point; we have not demonstrated that the dietary modifications we recommend will yield the dividends expected. We would point out to those people that the diet we eat today was not planned or developed for any particular purpose. It is a happenstance related to our affluence, the productivity of our farmers and the activities of our food industry. The risks associated with eating this diet are demonstrably large. The question to be asked, therefore, is not why should we change our diet but why not? What are the risks associated with eating less meat, less fat, less saturated fat, less cholesterol, less sugar, less salt, and more fruits, vegetables, unsaturated fat and cereal products—especially whole grain cereals. There are none that can be identified and important benefits can be expected.

Ischemic heart disease, cancer, diabetes and hypertension are the diseases that kill us. They are epidemic in our population. We cannot afford to temporize. We have an obligation to inform the public of the current state of knowledge and to assist the public in making the correct food choices. To do less is to avoid our responsibility.

Dr. Phillip Lee, Professor of Social Medicine and Director, Health Policy Program, University of California, San Francisco

The publication of *Dietary Goals for the United States* by the Senate Select Committee on Nutrition and Human Needs is a major step forward in the development of a rational national health policy. The public health problems related to what we eat are pointed out in *Dietary Goals*. More important, the steps that can and should be taken by individuals, families, educators, health professions, industry and Government are made clear.

As a Nation we have come to believe that medicine and medical technology can solve our major health problems. The role of such important factors as diet in cancer and heart disease has long been obscured by the emphasis on the conquest of these diseases through the miracles of modern medicine. Treatment not prevention, has been the order of the day.

The problems can never be solved merely by more and more medical care. The health of individuals and the health of the population is determined by a variety of biological (host), behavioral, sociocultural and environmental factors. None of these is more important than the food we eat. This simple fact and the importance of diet in health and disease is clearly recognized in *Dietary Goals for the United States*.

The Senate Select Committee on Nutrition and Human Needs has made four recommendations to encourage the achievement of the very sound dietary goals incorporated in the report. These are:

1. A large scale public nutrition education program involving the schools, food assistance programs, the Extension Service of the Department of Agriculture and the mass media.
2. Mandatory food labeling for all foods.

3. The development of improved food processing methods for institutional and home use.
4. Expanded federal support for research in human nutrition.

It is important that *Dietary Goals for the United States* be made widely available because it is the only publication of its kind and it will be an invaluable resource for parents, school teachers, public health nurses, health educators, nutritionists, physicians and others who are involved in providing people with information about the food they eat.

The recommendations, if acted upon promptly by the Congress, can help individuals, families and those responsible for institutional food services (schools, hospitals) be better informed about the consequences of present dietary habits and practices. Moreover, they provide a practical guide for action to improve the unhealthy situation that exists.

The effective implementation of the Senate Select Committee recommendations and the proposed dietary goals could have profound health and economic benefits. Not only would many people lead longer and healthier lives but the reduced burden of illness during the working lives of men and women would reduce the cost of medical care and increase productivity.

What can be done to assure sustained and effective action on these recommendations? First, the Congress can act to appropriate the needed funds for the proposed programs. In some instances, such as mandatory food labeling, it must also enact the authorizing legislation. Second, the new Secretaries of Agriculture and Health Education, and Welfare can act as soon as they take office to create a joint policy committee to address the issues raised by the Senate Select Committee and provide a means to assure that health considerations will no longer take a back seat to economic considerations in our food and agriculture policies. Finally, our greatest bulwark against the interests that have helped to create the present problems is an informed public.

Dr. Beverly Winikoff, Rockefeller Foundation, New York

What are the implications of these dietary goals?

The fact that the goals can be stated in nutritional terms first and then mirrored in a set of behavioral changes impels a closer look at why Americans eat the way they do. What people eat is affected not only by what scientists know, or by what doctors tell them, or even by what they themselves understand. It is affected by Government decisions in the area of agricultural policy, economic and tax policy, export and import policy, and involves questions of good production, transportation, processing, marketing, consumer choice, income and education, as well as food availability and palatability. Nutrition, then, is the end result of pushes and pulls in many directions, a response to the multiple forces creating the "national nutrition environment."

Even "personal dietary preferences" are not immutable but interact with other forces in the environment and are influenced by them. People learn the patterns of their diet not only from the family and its sociocultural background, but from what is available in the marketplace and what is promoted both formally through advertising and informally through general availability in schools, restaurants, supermarkets, work places, airports, and so forth.

It is generally recognized with regard to the overall economic climate that both what the Government does do and what it does not do shape the arena in which other forces interact. This is also true with regard to nutrition. In determining the parameters of the socio-economic system, Government also determines the nature of the national buffet. Government policy, then, must be made with full awareness of this responsibility.

It is increasingly obvious that if new knowledge is to result in new behaviors then people must be able to act, without undue obstacles, in accordance with the information that they learn. The problem of education for health as it has been practiced is that it has been in isolation, not to say oblivion, of the real pressures, expectations, and norms of society which mold and constrain individual behavior. There must be some coordination between what people are taught to do and what they can do. Part of the responsibility for this coordination rests with the Government's evaluation and coordination of its own activities. Effective education must be accompanied by Government policies which make it easier, indeed likely, that an individual will change his or her life-style in accordance with the information offered.

At present, we see a situation in which the opposite is often the case. Nutrition and health education are offered at the same time as barrages of commercials for soft drinks, sugary snacks, high-fat foods, cigarettes and alcohol. We put candy machines in our schools, serve high fat lunches to our children, and place cigarette machines in our work places. The American marketplace provides easy access to sweet soft drinks, high-sugar cereals, candies, cakes, and high-fat beef, and more difficult access to foods likely to improve national nutritional health.

This trend can be reversed by specific agricultural policies, pricing policies, and marketing policies, as well as the recommendations outlined in these "Dietary Goals for the United States."

In general, Americans have quite accurate perceptions of sound nutritional principles, as was demonstrated recently by a Harris poll conducted for the Mount Sinai Hospital in Chicago. However, people do lack understanding of the consequences of nutrition-related diseases. There is a widespread and unfounded confidence in the ability of medical science to cure or mitigate the effects of such diseases once they occur. Appropriate public education must emphasize the unfortunate but clear limitations of current medical practice in curing the common killing diseases. Once hypertension, diabetes, arteriosclerosis or heart disease are manifest, there is, in reality, very little that medical science can do to return a patient to normal physiological function. As awareness of this limitation increases, the importance of prevention will become all the more obvious.

But prevention is not possible solely through medical interventions. It is the responsibility of Government at all levels to take the initiative in creating for Americans an appropriate nutritional atmosphere—one conductive to improvement in the health and quality of life of the American people.

Data on the Relationship between Diet and Heart Disease

Coronary heart disease in all of its manifestations is the modern epidemic. Data from studies across the nation show that every fifth man and every seventeenth woman will have developed or died from coronary heart disease by age sixty. Coronary heart disease currently accounts for one-half of all deaths in the United States. Over one million Americans will have heart attacks this year, and two-thirds of these people will die as a result. The impact of heart disease on the health of the nation can be measured not only in terms of morbidity and mortality, but also in economic terms: direct costs of cardio-vascular disease have been estimated at $26.7 billion for 1977.

The pathological process underlying the vast majority of coronary heart disease and stroke episodes in Western nations is the development of atherosclerosis, the deposition of cholesterol-laden fatty plaques in blood vessels. Atherosclerosis results in narrowing of the arterial lumen, restricting the supply of oxygen to the affected tissue. Thus, atherosclerosis in the coronary arteries can lead to heart attacks (also called myocardial infarction), in the cerebral arteries to stroke, and in the renal arteries to kidney failure.

While the exact mechanism underlying atherogenesis—the development of these plaques—is not clearly understood, it has been hypothesized that the basic process involves injury to the endothelial cells lining the arterial walls, followed by a pouring of blood fats through this injury to lodge in the intimal space within the vessel wall. Fibrous growth may occur, resulting in the fibrous fatty plaque typical of atherosclerosis.

Many different factors can apparently lead to the initial injury of the endothelial cells. These range from high blood lipids, high blood pressure, or carboxyhemoglobin from cigarette smoke, to bacterial infections and auto-immune disorders. Because of this, it has been suggested that blood vessel injury may occur throughout the world. But in the less developed countries, this injury will usually be repaired with little or no harmful effects. It is apparently only in those nations whose populations typically have high blood lipids that atherosclerosis develops. This disease is so widespread in Western nations such as the United States that 48 percent of males in their early twenties already have evidence of atherosclerosis.[9]

The Role of Serum Cholesterol

The importance of high blood lipids—specifically serum cholesterol—in the development of atherosclerosis has been demonstrated beyond any reasonable doubt by many studies. The Framingham study, a prospective epidemiological study which has followed approximately five thousand men and women for over three decades, has established serum cholesterol level as one of the three most powerful risk indicators for subsequent cardio-

[9] McNamara JJ; Molot MA; Stremple JT, et al. "Coronary artery disease in combat causalities in Vietnam." J. Am. Assoc. *216*: 1185, 1971.

vascular disease, the other two being blood pressure and cigarette smoking.[10] For example, the incidence of coronary heart disease among males was over four times greater among those with cholesterol levels above 260 mg/dl than among those with cholesterol levels below 200 mg/dl.

This relationship of increasing risk of coronary heart disease with increasing serum cholesterol level has been corroborated in studies in Albany, Minneapolis, and elsewhere throughout the United States and the world. One landmark study in this respect was the Seven Countries study[11] which followed over 12,000 men in different locations in Europe, the United States and Japan. The international cross-cultural comparisons again clearly show a close relationship between serum cholesterol level and coronary heart disease incidence.

Can serum cholesterol levels be modified to decrease the coronary heart disease epidemic? The Seven Countries study has shown a strong correlation between dietary fat and serum cholesterol level. A strong correlation between dietary saturated fat and coronary heart disease death, and between dietary saturated fat and coronary heart disease incidence has also been demonstrated, leading support to the hypothesis that diet can influence risk of heart disease by altering serum cholesterol levels.

Diet and Serum Cholesterol

Many studies have in fact examined the effect of diet and its ability to raise or lower serum cholesterol levels. Because of the role of serum cholesterol and the nature of the fatty deposits of atherosclerosis, the dietary focus has primarily been on the effect of dietary fats and dietary cholesterol. In this regard, two studies often cited are those of Keys and co-workers,[12] and of Hegsted and co-workers.[13]

These studies consist of metabolic ward trials in which type of fat and amount of cholesterol were altered in the diets of persons under close observation. With each dietary change, the subsequent change in serum cholesterol level was noted. In these experiments, it was found that saturated fats such as those contained in coconut oil raise serum cholesterol levels, while polyunsaturated fats such as those that predominate in most vegetable oils lower serum cholesterol levels. Dietary cholesterol was found to have an effect independent of dietary fat on raising serum cholesterol.

Investigation of non-Western or non-industrialized countries and societies also reveals a striking lack of elevated cholesterol levels and low coronary heart disease morbidity and mortality. Generally, the people in these countries also consume diets very high in complex carbohydrates, and very low in animal foods and refined sugars. A review of data from the People's Republic of China, a country with low cardiovascular disease rates, reported that the average serum cholesterol level of the population was 136 mg/dl in normal subjects, and 190 mg/dl in coronary heart disease patients.[14] This compares

---

[10] Dawber TR. *The Framingham Study: The Epidemiology of Atherosclerotic Disease*. Cambridge, Mass.: Harvard University Press, 1980.

[11] Keys A. *Seven Countries: A Multivariate Analysis of Death and Coronary Heart Disease*. Cambridge, Mass: Harvard University Press, 1980.

[12] Keys A; Anderson JT; Grande F. "Serum cholesterol response to changes in the diet. I-IV. Metabolism." *14*: 747–787, 1965.

[13] Hegsted DM; McGandy RB; Myers ML; Stare FJ. "Quantitative effects of dietary fat on serum cholesterol in man." Am. J. Clin. Nutr. *17* (11): 281–295, 1965.

[14] Van die Redaskie. "Coronary heart disease in China." South African Med. J. *47*: 1485, 1973.

with an average value for Americans of approximately 220 mg/dl. Even in six-year-old American children, serum cholesterol levels may average close to 190 mg/dl,[15] a level which would put these children at higher than average risk of coronary heart disease in China.

The Tarahumara Indians of Mexico, known for their long kickball games, also have very low serum cholesterol levels, averaging 125 mg/dl.[16] A dietary investigation of the Tarahumaras revealed very low consumption of animal foods, the intake of which was highly correlated with serum cholesterol levels (Table 9). This study was significant in that

Table 9 Correlations Between the Plasma Cholesterol Concentration of the Tarahumara Indians and the Intakes of Certain Foods and Dietary Substances.*

Positive correlations ($P5$ 0.01)	
Cholesterol	0.898
Animal fat	0.593
Total fat	0.552
Eggs	0.548
Animal protein	0.464
Sugar	0.323
No correlations ($P5$ 0.01)	
Starch	0.145
Total calories	0.064
Plant sterols	0.030
Negative correlations ($P5$ 0.01)	
Vegetable protein	−0.723
Vegetable fat	−0.403
Fiber	−0.384

*Correlation coefficients were measured for a subsample of 103 adults (excluding pregnant and lactating women).

The correlation between the total plasma choleterol and dietary cholesterol intake per day (r=0.898, $P5$ 0.01) in a subsample of the Tarahumara study.

it was one of the first studies to demonstrate a strong correlation between individual dietary intake levels and individual serum cholesterol levels in a free-living population. This correlation has usually been difficult to observe because of the large amount of individual variation in food intake from day to day.

Perhaps the most interesting of these cross-cultural comparisons are the investigations comparing Japanese in Japan with Japanese in Hawaii and in California.[17] As with all

---

[15] Crawford PB; Clark MJ; Pearson RL; Huenemann RL. "Serum cholesterol of 6-year-olds in relation to environmental factors." J. Am. Diet. Assoc. *78*(1): 41–46, 1981.

[16] Connor WE; Cerqueria MT; Connor RW, et al. "The plasma lipids, lipoproteins, and diet of the Tarahumara Indians of Mexico." Am. J. Clin. Nutr. *31*(7): 1131–1142, July 1978.

[17] Kato H; Tillotson J; Nichaman MZ, et al. "Epidemiologic studies of coronary heart disease and stroke in Japanese men living in Japan, Hawaii and California: Serum lipids and diet." Am. J. Epidemiol. *97*(6): 372–385, 1973. Robertson TL; Kato H; Rhoads GG, et al. "Epidemiologic studies of coronary heart disease and stroke in Japanese men living in Japan, Hawaii and California: Incidence of myocardial infarction and death from coronary heart disease." Am J. Cardiol. *39* (2): 239–243, Feb. 1977.

Table 10 Comparisons between Japanese Men in Japan, Hawaii and California

Variable	Japan	Hawaii	California
Myocardial infarction incidence and coronary heart disease mortality	1.4	3.0	
(cases/1,000 person-yrs)		2.8	4.3
Serum cholesterol (mg/dl)	181.1±38.5*	218.3±38.2	228.2±42.2
Dietary variables (daily intake)			
Total fat (g)	36.6±20.4	85.1±38.9	94.8±36.4
Saturated fat (g)	16.0±13.3	59.1±32.7	66.3±30.5
Cholesterol (mg)	464.1±324.4	545.1±316.4	533.2±297.8
Simple carbohydrate (g)	61.1±37.4	91.6±54.7	96.4±53.9
Complex carbohydrate (g)	278.2±104.4	168.7±73.7	154.9±66.1
% calories from carbohydrate	15.1±6.9	33.3±9.4	37.5±8.1
% calories from carbohydrate	63.0±11.2	46.4±11.0	44.2±9.4

*Values are mean ± standard deviation.
(Adapted from Robertson, et al. and Kato, et al.)

migrant studies, these comparisons have the advantage of comparing genetically similar groups of people—in this case, all of Japanese ancestry—in different environments. Additionally, since Japan is a highly industrialized country, similar in this respect to the United States, inferences from differences in diet between these three groups can be made with more than the usual confidence. As can be seen in Table 10, the trends in comparing these three populations has shown that the Japanese in Japan eat much less fat and saturated fat, and much more complex carbohydrate than in California, with Hawaiian intakes falling between the two. This also held true for serum cholesterol levels and coronary heart disease mortality, both of which were significantly related to dietary variables.

Examination of groups within industrialized societies with differing dietary habits also have shown a relationship between diet, serum cholesterol, and coronary heart disease mortality. Among the most investigated of these groups are the Seventh-Day Adventists[18]. It has been consistently observed that the vegetarians among the Seventh-Day Adventists have lower serum cholesterol levels than the omnivores among this religious group. As a whole, Seventh-Day Adventists also have lower serum cholesterol levels than the general United States population, demonstrating that other factors in their life-style also decrease their coronary heart disease risk. A recently published report of a six-year prospective study also showed that Seventh-Day Adventists living in California have lower coronary heart disease mortality rates than their fellow Californians. This decreased mortality was lower for the vegetarians than the non-vegetarians, significantly so in males.

Although these studies have all pointed toward a strong link between diet and coronary heart disease, none of the above studies have actually tried to alter a person's diet to see if that will lead to lower serum cholesterol levels and eventually decrease coronary heart disease morbidity and mortality. There have in fact been several clinical trials,

---

[18] West RO; Hayes OB. "Diet and serum cholesterol levels: A comparison between vegetarians and nonvegetarians in a Seventh-Day Adventist group." Am. J. Clin. Nutr. *21*(8): 853–862, Aug. 1968. Phillips RL; Lemon FR; Beeson WL; Kuzma JW. "Coronary heart disease mortality among Seventh-Day Adventists with differing dietary habits: A primary report." Am. J. Clin. Nutr. *31*(10): S191–S198, Oct. 1978.

often with persons having very high risk for coronary heart disease, which have attempted to do just that.

Clinical Trials

Generally, these clinical trials have been classically designed, with two study groups, one given explicit instructions to change their dietary habits in the hope of preventing coronary heart disease, the other a control group, without the dietary counseling. After following these study groups for a number of years, differences between the groups in endpoints such as the proportion of coronary heart disease death and heart attack rate have been compared.

The first major clinical trial was the so-called "Anti-Coronary Club" trial, started in 1957 by the Bureau of Nutrition of the New York City Department of Health.[19] It was for this study that the "Prudent Diet" was conceived, a diet with emphasis on increasing polyunsaturated fat in the diet, and decreasing total fat, saturated and cholesterol, not unlike the guidelines now known as the U.S. Dietary Goals.

During the course of the study, serum cholesterol levels in the group that actively followed the diet were lowered significantly relative to the control group (Table 11).[20]

Table 11 Fifteen-year Follow-up in the Anti-Coronary Club Trial

Variable	Active diet group	Inactive diet group	Control
40–49 years			
Number with hypercholesterolemia*, % change	−50.0	−24.9	−5.9
Coronary heart disease incidence, cases/1,000 person-yrs	4.65**	12.82	7.84
50–59 years			
Number with hypercholesterolemia, % change	−44.5	−27.4	−13.5
Coronary heart disease incidence, cases/1,000 person-yrs	13.09**	18.24	20.10

*Hypercholesterolemia = serum cholesterol $\geq$ 260 mg/dl
**Significantly different from cholesterol, $p < 0.05$
(Adapted from Singman, et al.)

After fifteen years of follow-up, the incidence of coronary heart disease in the diet group was two-thirds that of the control group. A similar dietary approach was prescribed in the Los Angeless Veterans Administration study,[21] and again, after eight years of follow-up, the diet group had significantly less atherosclerotic events—sudden death, heart

---

[19] Christakis G; Rinzler SH; Archer M, et al. "The Anti-Coronary Club: A dietary approach to the prevention of coronary heart disease." A seven-year report. Am. J. Publ. Health *56*(2): 299–314, Feb. 1966.

[20] Singman HS; Berman SN; Cowell C, et al. "The Anti-Coronary Club: 1957 to 1972." Am. J. Clin. Nutr. *33*(6): 1183–1191, June 1980.

[21] Dayton S; Pearce ML. "Prevention of coronary heart disease and other complications of atherosclerosis by modified diet." Am. J. Med. *46*: 751–762, May 1969. Dayton S; Pearce ML; Hashimoto S, et al. "A clinical trial of high unsaturated fat diet." Circulation 39–40 (Suppl. 2): 1, July 1969.

Table 12   The Los Angeles Veterans Administration Study: Eight-Year Follow-up

	Diet	Control	P
Number of men	424	422	
Fatal atherosclerotic events	48	70	0.05
Fatal and non-fatal atherosclerotic events	66	96	0.01
Any definite or possible atherosclerotic event	110	136	0.05

(Adapted from Dayton & Pearce.)

Table 13   The Oslo Diet-heart Study: Eleven-year Mortality

Manifestation	Diet	Control	P
Fatal myocardial infarction	32	57	0.004
Total sudden deaths	52	53	—
Total coronary heart disease mortality	79	94	0.097
Total cardiovascular mortality	88	102	0.13
Total mortality	101	108	—
Serum cholesterol at 5 years	244	285	
% decrease from initial value	17.6	3.7	

(Adapted from Leren.)

attack, or stroke—than the control group (Table 12). The diet group also had serum cholesterol levels 12.7 percent lower than the control group.

While the Anti-Coronary Club and Los Angeles Veterans Administration studies were aimed at primary prevention of atherosclerotic disease, another trial of diet and heart disease, the Oslo Diet-Heart study,[22] was aimed at secondary prevention. Thus, the study population consisted of patients with past history of heart trouble who were then followed for eleven years. Again, serum cholesterol levels in the diet group were significantly lower than that of the control group, as was the number of fatal heart attacks (Table 13). However, there was virtually no difference in total mortality between the two groups. The same effect was reported in the Finnish Mental Hospital Study,[23] in which one hospital was given a serum cholesterol lowering diet, while another hospital served as the control group (Table 14).

Unfortunately, these clinical trials have failed to be very dramatic in their effect, leading skeptics to claim that dietary prevention of heart disease has yet to be demonstrated conclusively and therefore may not be possible. However, there are two simple reasons that the effect has not been strong. The first of these is that the dietary changes were minor—it could be argued that it is remarkable that significant differences were observed with such small dietary changes. One can only speculate what might have been observed if the diet group had eaten macrobiotically rather than followed variations of the Prudent Diet. The other reason is that in these studies, the diet groups still had average serum cholesterol levels above that which is average for Americans—a level

[22] Leren P. "The Oslo Diet-Heart study." Eleven-year report. Circulation 42: 935–942, Nov. 1970.
[23] Miettinen M; Turpeinen O; Karvonen MJ, et al. "Effect of cholesterol-lowering diet on mortality from coronary heart disease and other causes: A twelve-year clinical trial in men and women." Lancet 2: 835–838, 21 Oct. 1972.

Table 14   Mortality in the Finnish Mental Hospital Study

Cause	*men*		*women*	
	Diet	Control	Diet	Control
Coronary heart disease	6.61*	14.08	5.21	7.90
Cerebrovascular disease	1.74	2.42	2.23	2.02
Other cardiovascular disease	3.18	2.47	3.14	2.40
Cancer	5.02	3.96	4.08	3.72
All diseases	32.00	35.96	29.05	27.21
All causes	34.84	39.50	30.87	29.01

*Significantly different from control, $p=0.05$
(Adapted from Miettinen, et al.)

which still leads to an atheroslcerosis epidemic. Thus, the experience of the diet groups could not begin to approach the experiences of vegetarians or non-Western societies.

The dietary groups were still galloping toward atherosclerosis; they only were galloping at slightly slower speeds than the controls.

Therefore, interpretation of these studies needs to be made in the context of the whole of cardiovascular research. While any one these studies has questionable significance, they have all demonstrated an impact on coronary heart disease incidence and mortality. That the impact has been in the direction predicted by other studies reinforces the conclusion that, in the aggregate, these trials are convincing evidence for the important role of diet in the prevention of coronary heart disease.

Lawrence H. Kushi

Chapter 4

Macrobiotics, Preventive Medicine, and Society

New Directions in Modern Medicine

Robert S. Mendelsohn, M.D.

I would like to review several of the more positive changes that have taken place in modern medicine over the last several years, as well as several medically related developments within society at large. Based on these and similar trends, I would also like to offer a number of predictions about the future.

There have been at least eight major advances in the last several years:

1. In 1980, the American Medical Association came out against the routine annual physical examination. I consider this to be a major breakthrough. The annual physical examination has been, until now, one of the major rituals in modern medicine. It has existed since the Great Depression when doctors did not have enough business, so they decided that everyone should have an examination every year. They were quickly followed by dentists, and both groups rapidly turned to x-rays.

   The routine physical examination has become so counterproductive that the AMA had to come out against it. When I heard this, I thought that they must have read my book, *Confessions of a Medical Heretic*, because the chapter that deals with the annual physical examination is entitled, "If This Is Preventive Medicine, I'll Take My Chances with Disease." My prediction is that now that the routine annual physical examination (and their x-rays) is being prescribed, the incidence of cancer will certainly drop. So I am very happy to see the AMA come out against the routine physical examination.

2. Also in 1980, the American Cancer Society came out against the routine annual chest x-ray. Now when I saw that happen, I could hardly believe it. I could not believe that modern medicine could move so fast in one year. I think it is quite clear that x-rays play a part in the causation of cancer. We know that mammography, used to detect breast cancer, can certainly cause breast cancer, and I do not think there is any question that now that we are getting rid of the annual examination of the chest by x-ray, the incidence of cancer is going to go down.

3. In that same year, the American Cancer Society came out against the routine annual Pap smear, and that interested me because the incidence of error in the Pap smear is somewhere between 20 percent and 30 percent. Also, there is no evidence, throughout the two decades that the Pap smear has been in existence, of any change in the mortality or incidence of cervical cancer between areas where the Pap smear is extensively used and areas where it is not used at all. Since the error rate is so high, my prediction is that the dropping of the routine annual Pap smear will also result in a drop in the rate of cancer.

4. In 1980, sales of Valium dropped by 30 percent. Now I do not want to take the credit for that, even though I am willing to take the credit; because I always take credit for things I do not deserve to make up for the blame for things I do not deserve. But in this case, I have to give credit to a woman who wrote a book called *I'm Dancing As Fast As I Can*. Her name is Barbara Gordon. The book tells how to get off of Valium, which doctors do not know how to tell you. Doctors tell you how to get on drugs. But they do not tell you how to get off.

5. The national tripling of home births is my next area of praise. This has surprised me because I never thought that so many people would opt out of the temple of modern medicine and decide to carry out the sacrament of birth at home instead of in a hospital. Because, as you know, modern medicine likes you to carry out the sacrament of birth and the sacrament of death inside the temple; in both cases this works at destroying your family. Recently obstetricians will allow you to have your husband with you, but they still snatch away the baby and put him or her into a newborn nursery.

   At the other end of life, of course, you have to die under conditions of intensive care where the visiting hours are five minutes out of every hour, and you have 55 minutes to die with no family or friends around; where there is only a monitor to hear your last words. (I come from a generation where the word "monitor" meant "hallguard," and I still have trouble with that word.)

6. The next advance is the recent recommendation of the National Institutes of Health against automatic repeat Caesarian sections and against automatic sections for breech babies. Now that surprised me because as most of you know, the incidence of sections has risen from a normal rate of 4 percent or 5 percent to somewhere between 20 percent and 40 percent. And in large research and teaching hospitals, some of which are in Boston, the rates have been found to be over 50 percent. That is due to the mistaken notion that "once a section always a section." I thought it would take over twenty years before we could get rid of what I call "the old doctor's tale." Recently, I debated on television with George Ryan, M.D., who is the incoming president of the American College of Obstetrics and Gynecology. He said on television that doctors were already giving up automatic repeat sections and automatic sections for breech babies. (One of the cardinal beliefs of modern medicine is that God made a mistake when He did not put a zipper in every woman's belly.) Obstetricians in general believe that the best way to have a baby is by Caesarian section, but they do not say exactly that. They turn to religious terms. As an example, they often say "Would you not rather have your baby from above than below?" And since the expression "from above" has the aura of divinity about it, who wants to have a baby from below?

7. The next advance is the action of my own organization, the American Academy of Pediatrics, endorsing breastfeeding; only twenty-three years behind the La Leche League. This action also violates one of the beliefs of modern medicine, since pediatricians have always felt that God made a mistake when He did not put Similac in women's breasts. But now they are en-

dorsing breastfeeding and the incidence has risen in this country from 15 percent in the 1960's to a present rate of 63 percent. I predict that soon infant formula will finally be recognized as the "granddaddy of all junk food."
8. The next advance is the 1980 Food and Drug Administration action to remove three thousand drugs from the market. I do not know how many of you saw that in your paper. It was in the *Washington Post.*

These are eight major advances in modern medicine which I think will mark a turnaround. Now all of modern medicine is beginning to backpedal as quickly as it possibly can. It is even beginning to take credit for the drop in cancer incidence and mortality that I predict will happen. And I am perfectly happy to give them credit. For as far as I can tell, as soon as doctors stop practicing the kind of medicine they have been practicing over the last forty years, the incidence of cancer is bound to go down.

Now I want to give you some idea what has happened inside of medicine, because some of you might not have had the opportunity to keep up with all the recent medical journals. One of the studies that I have been quoting for a long time is twelve years old. It comes from a book by two British doctors, named, appropriately enough, Sharp and Keene. The name of the book is *Presymptomatic Detection and Early Diagnosis.* This study, done in England, showed that the Pap smear was valueless, and that there was no difference in the incidence or mortality in those who used the Pap smear and those who did not.

The same study was repeated last year by two doctors from New York University and Yale. The doctor from New York is Dr. Annemarie Foltz, and the one from Yale is Jennifer L. Kelsey. They pointed out that it has not been well established that the screening of large numbers of women has had any effect on the death rate from cervical cancer. Questioning the current medical practice of the yearly Pap smear on adult women, these researchers state that there is a 20–30 percent incidence of false negatives found, to say nothing of the incidence of false positives. They point out the questionable accuracy of the test, and also the fact that it became standard recommended policy without ever having been subjected to controlled trials to determine its efficacy.

The next item is from Francis Straus, Professor of Pathology, at my own University of Chicago. Dr. Straus pointed out the technical problem associated with biopsies. I want to quote several sentences which describe things that can go wrong. This is from a publication *Cancer News for Physicians,* published in the fall of 1979. As Dr. Straus points out, once the biopsy sample has been delicately removed from the patient, it is not out of danger. It is all too easy to lay the biopsy down on a sterile prep tray (if you have ever stood in an operating room, you might know exactly how true this is), or to become engrossed in repairing a surgical defect while the tiny morsel desiccates into a tiny unrecoverable shadow of its former self, compressed by distortion from repeated picking up by forceps' teeth or squeezing through fingertips. I cannot tell you how often I have seen this, especially in research and teaching hospitals where everybody has to squeeze that biopsy to feel if it is soft or hard. (This also happens to women in labor, as everyone has to come in and do a vaginal examination—intern, resident doctor, nurse, cleaning lady, etc.)

Dr. Straus continues to caution us—i.e., one important but often overlooked aspect of performing a biopsy is the cleanliness and sharpness of the biopsy instrument. Frequently the biopsy tool contains tissue fragments from the previous biopsy which dry and later are autoclaved with the instrument. Such desiccated particles impair the function of the instrument and confuse the pathologist (all we need is a confused pathologist) when mixed with the current specimen. Many cup forceps biopsies are torn off, because the cutting edge of the instrument has been allowed to become blunted through continual use.

The next is item from John Gofman, M.D., Ph.D., an expert on leukemia. Dr. Gofman points out that each year dental and medical diagnostic x-rays are responsible for 12,000 extra fatal cancers. He also points out that when the technician takes the x-ray, as many as one extra film per three is common—only taken to correct for errors. And for those of you who are interested in sexism and medicine, watch who goes in to take the x-rays and then watch who reads the x-rays. In my experience, it is almost always the male doctors who sit in their office and read the x-rays, while the female technician actually takes them.

Arthur Upton, former director of the National Cancer Institute, pointed out the risk of x-rays to radiologists, including a strong association with leukemia, skin cancer, lymphoma, and cancer of the brain. I always knew that radiologists had a higher incidence of leukemia, but I did not know they also had these other diseases. X-ray treatment for arthritis of the spine can produce an increased risk of cancer of the pancreas, leukemia, and other neoplasms. At the same time, studies on pregnant women have revealed that prenatal exposure to x-rays involving a dose on the order of one rad (that is what you get from one chest x-ray or from a full-mouth dental x-ray) is associated with a 50 percent increase in the risk of childhood leukemia. According to the *British Medical Journal*, children born to hospital anesthetists are sixty times more likely to suffer from cancer than other children. The incidence of breast cancer in women anesthetists was also found to be fifty times higher than normal. Exposure to anesthetics can cause problems ranging from cleft lips and cleft palates to severe neurologic difficulties, bone and muscle disorders, impaired intellectual development, a low birth rate, and a higher incidence of miscarriage among anesthetists. Thirty percent of the anesthetists studied had problems getting pregnant.

Every once in a while a treatment for cancer comes out that is claimed to be perfectly safe. I am used to that, because one of the rules in medicine is to always use a new drug as quickly as you can before the side effects become known. So, for example, these days, ultra-sound, amniocentesis and bilirubin lights are being extensively used, even though we already know the dangers of those procedures. Vasectomy is another procedure which is still used extensively (over a million operations a year) even though the dangers of vasectomy are already known.

As far as cancer is concerned, a new drug came out a few years ago called Tamoxifen, which is used in certain cases of cancer of the breast. Here is the latest description of its side effects. This drug might produce oncogenic activity in animals. For those of you who do not know Greek, oncogenic means tumor-producing. I am very interested in chemotherapeutic agents causing cancer, because Interferon, which I am sure you are going to hear more about, comes in four types. One type, Lymphoblastoid Interferon, can cause cancer according to the press release sent out by Searle Laboratories. I did not see one newspaper pick that up. So now if your doctor wants to give you Interferon, ask him which kind.

The next item is from *Lancet*, March 15, 1980. This prestigious medical journal reports that the overall survival rate of patients with primary breast cancer has not improved in the last ten years despite increasing use of multiple drug chemotherapy for treatment of metastases. Furthermore, there has been no improvement in survival from the first metastasis, and survival might have even been shortened in some patients given chemotherapy.

Many patients come to me because they want to know whether or not they should go for chemotherapy. My answer is always to ask your doctor whether he has any study on patients who have refused chemotherapy. The doctor will probably tell you they have no studies because they do not follow up on those patients. However, he will probably tell you that they have an 80 percent cure rate on those they do follow up on. My answer to that is "how do you know that the other group does not have a 90 percent cure rate?" But if you want to, you can always take up the *Lancet* article with your doctor, although I warn you to be careful, because your doctor might fire you. This is one of those strange financial interactions in life where the employee can fire the employer. If he does not actually dismiss you as a patient, the doctor might get angry with you, because there are only two things that doctors do not like to hear from patients. I owe this line to David Stewart, Ph.D., who is head of NAPSAC (National Association of Parents and Professionals for Safe Alternatives in Childbirth), who says that the only things doctors do not like to hear are: (1) something they already know, and (2) something they do not know. Otherwise, they are always ready to listen to anything as long as it does not take too long.

I am now going to go on to my predictions. My first prediction is that more and more people are going to be turning to alternative systems. I cannot tell you strongly enough how grateful I am to Mr. Kushi and associates for introducing me to macrobiotics as something I can offer my patients. The macrobiotic movement, which once was regarded as out of the mainstream, has now become very mainstream as a result of the activities of the Senate Nutrition Committee, as well as meetings such as those held by Michio Kushi and the East West Foundation in Washington (refer to Mr. Kushi's introduction in Chapter 1).

Macrobiotics, and other similar nutritional approaches, are going to gain increasingly large audiences. However, macrobiotics in particular has several distinct advantages which guarantee it an ever-ascending place in American society. I predict that in several years, the AMA is going to say that the reason why the rate of cancer has diminished is because of their activities such as those mentioned earlier in this presentation. We are going to claim that the cancer rate went down because the nutritional habits of the people have changed. Both sides are right.

In conclusion, let me present three ways in which macrobiotics is different from conventional nutritional science:

Number 1: Macrobiotics appreciates and emphasizes the crucial importance of societal, cultural and familial background in determining proper dietary patterns. I think that this is crucial in understanding that diet is only part of the whole.

Number 2: Macrobiotics appreciates and emphasizes the crucial importance of prenatal nutrition and breastfeeding in determining the future development of each individual. I think that this is very important because the other systems that I have looked at do not emphasize strongly enough the effect of prenatal and infant nutrition.

Number 3: Macrobiotics appreciates and emphasizes the crucial importance of incorporating diet into a universal system of thought and behavior. It does not get caught in the trap of singling out cholesterol or vitamins or trace minerals or protein. Macrobiotics is a synthesizing system. American nutrition in contrast depends on analysis. Some of you who are interested in psychiatry might remember one of the rules of psychiatry which states that after your patient has spent enough time in analysis, he develops a state of inaction known as "paralysis through analysis."

My final prediction is that cancer will eventually be conquered, not through surgery, x-ray treatments or chemotherapy—not even by Laetrile. Cancer will be conquered by the profound wisdom of leaders like Michio Kushi and universal truths like macrobiotics.

Macrobiotics and Preventive Health Care

Paul Schulman

The overriding issue facing the health care profession in the United States, as well as the rest of the world, is the escalating cost of providing acute and chronic care for a population that is increasingly suffering from illness as a result of poor diet, inadequate exercise, and not living in harmony with nature.[1]

The increasing emphasis on acute and chronic care stems from a number of factors, including the ability, through technological and scientific advances, to provide life support systems, medications, and other modalities which serve to ameliorate the immediate symptoms of disease. Treatment is emphasized rather than finding the cause of or preventing disease. This orientation is in turn related to the general Western view of trying to conquer nature rather than attempting to live in harmony with it.

There is now a great deal of lip service being given to the issue of holding down costs, but there has been little direct action aimed at promoting health or at developing a budget for health promotion. For example, less than 1 percent of the federal budget for health care is presently dedicated to preventive programs or to promoting good health.[2]

---

[1] In 1979, total payments to doctors and hospitals in the United States averaged $3,500 for a family of four. The total cost of medical treatment in the United States was approximately $206 billion, an increase of 429 percent over the $38.9 billion spent in 1965. In July, 1982 the U.S. Government reported that medical spending increased 15.1 percent during 1981, reaching a total of nearly $287 billion, not counting research and construction expenditures. This accounts for nearly 9.8 percent of the American economy's total output of goods and services—the highest share in U.S. history. On a per-capita basis, national medical expenditures became a thousand dollar item for the first time in 1980—increasing by more than 14 percent to $1075. The 1981 increase to $1225 added another 14.9 percent, and government officials reported that the trend in 1982 has been so far the same.

The 15.1 percent increase in 1981 is twice the general rate of inflation and the cost of certain elements within the overall total rose by more than this amount: for example, the cost of hospital treatment increased by 17.5 percent to $118 billion and the bill for doctors' services rose by 16.9 percent to $55 billion. At the persent rate of increase, it is estimated that medical costs will double every five years, reaching over $400 billion by 1984. The American Heart Association has estimated that the United States could save at least $40 billion annually in medical costs through the widespread adoption of a preventive nutritional approach.

[2] Despite the substantial evidence linking diet to both the cause and possible treatment of disease, surprisingly little of the tremendous amount spent for medical research has been channeled into further studies of this relationship. For example, in fiscal 1979, the $13 million allocated by the National Cancer Institute represented only 1.8 percent of a research budget totalling over $743 million.

The geometric escalation of health care costs is related to two factors: the very high utilization of manpower in health care facilities, nursing homes, hospitals, and clinics, and increasing wages that are paid for those employees: and the increasing use of technology due to the fact that many people believe they can successfully attack illnesses by throwing money, equipment, and new technology at them. In actuality, the causes of those illnesses are fairly simple and could be ameliorated at a much lower cost or at no cost at all by a change in attitude and life-style. The Surgeon General's report for 1980 reviewed the fact that over 50 percent of all chronic illnesses are caused by poor nutrition, smoking, and the misuse of alcohol and other drugs, and that changes in attitudes and life-style could dramatically reduce both the incidences of mortality and morbidity among the general population and substantially reduce health care costs.[3]

The most essential components for maintaining health are (1) eating a diet that is very high in whole grains, naturally grown, organic foods, local vegetables, and other supplemental foods with very little or no meat and processed food: (2) a life-style based on daily and regular exercise: and (3) an attitude about wellness and health promotion that includes a desire to decrease smoking, drinking, and the ingestion of harmful toxic substances. In addition, an awareness of our relationship to each other and to the entire planet is essential.

Unfortunately, the medical profession has, until now, defined for itself a role which focuses on treating those patients who are the sickest and who need acute intervention. The medical profession has yet to view itself as model for the promotion of public health, and in many cases has contributed to the development of iatrogenic illnesses.[4] It has also been somewhat counter-productive in developing models that the general public can accept and use in order to make positive changes in attitudes and life-styles. The nursing profession, on the other hand, almost from its inception, has been much more concerned with health promotion and developing the life-styles and attitudes necessary for a healthy mind, body, and spirit.

However, a number of positive changes are also occurring at the present time.

---

[3] To date, at least eighteen health agencies throughout the world have issued reports which, like *Dietary Goals*, implicate diet as a major factor in the development of chronic disease and make dietary recommendations aimed at prevention. These include the USDA-HEW *Dietary Guidelines* issed in 1980, and the Surgeon General's *Report on Health Promotion and Disease Prevention* issued in 1979. The recommendations made by the Surgeon General, "people should consume . . . less saturated fat and cholesterol . . . less red meat . . . more complex carbohydrates such as whole grains, cereals, fruits, and vegetables" are typical of those made in these reports.
[4] Regarding nutrition education, for example, a recent article published by the Washington-based Center for Science in the Public Interest titled, *Diet and Health: A Missing Link in Your Doctor's Education*, mentions that according to an AMA survey, only thirty of the nation's 125 medical schools have required courses in nutrition, in spite of the increasing evidence that diet is a crucial factor in the prevention of sickness. In a report prepared by the U.S. Government Accounting Office, an AMA survey is again quoted as stating that "medical education and medical practices have not kept abreast of the tremendous advances in nutrition knowledge" and that "there is inadequate recognition, support, and attention given to this subject in medical schools."

The huge escalation in health care costs has forced both industry and government to begin reassessing what is happening in the medical profession. The development of health maintenance organizations, prepaid programs, and wellness programs both in industry and in many health care institutions are indicative of a change in attitude toward the current U.S. medical model. There has also been a shift in priorities among the general public. The development of exercise and fitness programs and their acceptance by the public as well as the general trend over the last few years toward less consumption of saturated, fatty foods indicate that the public is well ahead of many medical professionals and government leaders in acknowledging the need to change life-styles and attitudes in order to prevent illness. These are the types of changes that will create the motivating force which the medical profession will eventually follow.

Macrobiotics has at least two contributions to make in this area. The first is through the diet itself, which will result in improved health for those who begin to use it. The second will arise as those who have used the diet to achieve better health begin to spread this awareness to others. A good example of this occurred at the Shattuck Hospital in Boston when we introduced the macrobiotic diet to the staff. (The diet is now being introduced to the patients as well.) The project began as an overall wellness program which included exercise, meditation, and yoga. It was designed to help those on the medical, nursing, and support staffs who are under particular stress due to the continual need to make correct decisions concerning medications. The fact that Shattuck is a chronic illness facility where the prognosis for most of the patients is poor adds more stress. In addition, Shattuck is a state hospital, and many staff members tend to have lower self-esteem because state pay, fringe benefits, and career opportunities are usually less than in private institutions.

The wellness program was designed to increase the self-image of the staff while developing methods of coping with stress, and also to provide the staff with an opportunity to experience a new diet by introducing macrobiotic food to the hospital. About 50 percent of the staff members (approximately 500 employees) have chosen the macrobiotic food. For these, the impact of the diet has been very great, especially for those who were on medication and who have since been able to stop medication as a result of changing their diet and participating in other aspects of the program. (See Appendix.)

However, there have still been difficulties in initiating more detailed research into the specific benefits of the diet. First, there has not been, up until now, a strong desire on the part of medical staffs to apply for research protocols in the area of diet and nutrition, and secondly, there has not been a healthy supply of funds available from the federal government to support this kind of research. This is, however, beginning to change. Recent articles about the lower incidences of lung cancer in smokers who eat vegetables (see Appendix, Chapter 2) and the recent Department of Agriculture funding of the Tufts Nutrition Center are indicative of a change in priorities both among the medical profession and those in government who are responsible for allocating research dollars.

Among the many institutions which are adopting changes in their food service programs are prisons and other correctional institutions as the connection between a high sugar intake and other dietary factors and violent behavior becomes increasingly apparent. There is no question that we will begin to see, over the next several years, a tremendous increase in research on the relationship of diet and behavior.

If health care institutions in the United States hope to remain important to their communities, they must begin to recognize the need to promote health and optimal wellness in addition to treating acute illness, trauma, and chronic disease.

The inability of our current medical model to reduce the rates of cancer and heart disease and the increasing problems of mental illness, alcoholism, and drug abuse will eventually force both the public and the medical profession to reallocate their resources toward a preventive model which encourages self-responsibility in maintaining health. This new model will emerge very rapidly as economic resources continue to dry up through the 1980s.

In the future, I believe that we will see an increasing movement away from the present medical model and toward the integration of various modalities including acupuncture, body work, and macrobiotics. I forsee many health care institutions assuming the role of educational and training centers to provide the public with the means to maintain health.

A New Concept of Preventive Medicine

Richard Donze, D.O.

There is an old proverb which says that if you give a man a piece of bread, he can eat today, but if you teach him how to grow wheat, he can eat forever. Throughout this country, in the hospitals, clinics, and physicians' offices, there are scores of hungry people—the patients—and conventional medicine usually attempts to satisfy their hunger by giving them bread, lots of it. The bread business is really booming. Some people make a good living in it. Other people and their insurance companies spend a lot of money for it and keep coming back for more. What I am talking about is symptomatic medicine: the approach in which the main orientation is the elimination of symptoms, usually without eradicating the underlying cause and often ignoring it completely. Symptomatic medicine is a temporary solution to a problem that is either chronic or recurring, and it gives a false sense of security, analogous to turning off a fire alarm and believing that that action will put out the fire.

This approach is also known as "crisis intervention"—the situation in which people pay attention to their health only when they lose it, as in the old saying, "You don't know what you've got until it's gone."

When a health problem—an ache, a pain, a fever, an infection—develops, the afflicted person quickly runs to the doctor for help and says, "Doc, what can I do to make the pain go away," or "What can I do to make the infection go away?" The doctor then prescribes one or another magic potion or pill and usually the problem does disappear, because of, or more often, in spite of, the treatment that is given. And this goes on for much of a person's life: there is a crisis, but it is averted until the next one comes along, and so on and so on. Nobody worrys, because no matter what happens, the doctor can always fix it, and if he cannot fix it, he can always cut it out.

Then one day something terrible happens, something that a patient has seen happen to others time and time again but never really expected to happen to him. One day the problem is so big and so bad that the doctor cannot fix it anymore, and he cannot even cut it out.

Some of us realize that temporary solutions are just that—temporary. We know that there is a bottom to the doctor's black bag, and there is a limit to the number of magic rabbits that he can pull out of it. When that limit is reached, we as physicians have to tell the patient something he thought he would never hear. It is worse than telling him what is wrong with him. It is, "There is nothing else we can do. Go home and die or stay here in our hospital. We will put you to sleep until you die." And the patient feels cheated, disappointed by the one person or team of persons in whom he had really learned to put all of his confidence.

I think we expect so much of modern medicine because we were spoiled by its past successes and expect their repetition. Earlier in this century, medicine did or at least seemed to do some truly incredible things. For example, when scientists found the bacteria that were responsible for tuberculosis and pneumonia and the antibiotics that would kill those bacteria, suddenly the two major causes of death were curable. Even though it has been pointed out by many people that these diseases actually started to decline before the advent of antibiotics—largely through better sanitation and public health methods—their eradication is usually ascribed to the wonders of modern medicine.

But we have different problems facing us today. Instead of infectious diseases being the major cause of death, the so-called degenerative diseases have taken their place. Cardiovascular disease, or disease of the heart and blood vessels accounts for approximately 50 percent of all deaths in this country. Cancer claims another 20 percent. Many people today expect the same type of cures for these problems as there were for tuberculosis and pneumonia. They say, "Doc, keep me alive; maybe in another week, another month, there will be a breakthrough. Maybe they will find a cure." After all, the medical bulletins are always telling us that the answer to these riddles is just around the bend or right on the horizon.

Well, the dream is over and it is time for us to wake up. There probably is no cure as such for heart disease or cancer. We have been hearing "just around the bend" and "on the horizon" for a long time now, and not much has happened, except that more people have died.

Degenerative diseases seem to be multifaceted, with many different factors contributing to their existence, especially that of the individual's life-style. So how can there be one single cure? There is not and will not be one single magic bullet, be it chemotherapy, Laetrile, bypass surgery, vitamin C, Interferon, or even brown rice. It is time for us to wake up and grow up and to discard the image of doctors as surrogate mammies and daddies who know all the answers and who can always pick us up when we fall. We have to finally realize that the only way to cure degenerative diseases is not to get them in the first place. This is called prevention, and it is something each person must do by him or herself. Very few people realize this; very few people think they have any control over what happens to them.

During the years of my medical training and practice, I always found it interesting to observe the way people react when told they have a life-threatening illness such as heart disease or cancer. Many are depressed at their prospects; some become angry, but almost all exhibit surprise. They never believed it could happen to them. "Other people usually get these ailments—not me," they will say, and, "I don't understand how this could have happened. I haven't been sick a day in my life. Then suddenly, this." But these problems do not occur suddenly—they develop silently and insidiously.

This was demonstrated very clearly during the Korean and Vietnam wars when Army physicians performed autopsies on soldiers killed in action. They found significant degrees of arteriosclerosis—blood vessels choking with deposits of fat and cholesterol in men who were in their late teens and early twenties, in the physical prime of life. Yet it is reasonable to assume that had these soldiers lived they would later have developed some type of degenerative disease.

So there are probably many people today who are walking around with time bombs ticking away inside, waiting to explode; and when the explosion finally does occur, they will wonder where it came from. They will be surprised, because people tend to dissociate themselves from their illnesses. They do not realize that they themselves have a lot to do with why it occurred, that they actually set the bomb ticking. They think the problem happened *to* them, that it was imposed *on* them by some malevolent force in nature. They believe they had nothing to do with it, that they are simply victims in some unfair game of chance.

And with this victim mentality comes a sense of powerlessness, a sense of helplessness in which they believe they cannot change their unfortunate state, so they submit to me, the physician, and ask me to change things for them. Since they believe the problem originated outside of themselves, they believe it can only be taken away in the same manner, by someone or something outside of themselves.

Somewhere along the line, the idea came along that the way to beat degenerative disease is to find it early; to accomplish this, many people pay a visit to their doctor for a so-called routine checkup. This physical examination is often accompanied by blood tests and electro-cardiograms and sometimes by x-rays and other screening procedures. This practice is referred to as preventive medicine, but actually this is misleading. It is simply early detection; there is very little or no prevention involved. Many people feel comforted when they get a clean bill of health from the doctor, but this scheme is totally inadequate for the problems facing us today. Cardiovascular disease and cancer account for over 70 percent of all deaths that occur. When we find them it is usually too late. Once these problems become obvious to the medical practitioner, and we decide it is time to act, the futility of our actions is like closing the old gate after the horse got out. The most we can hope for is prolonging the inevitable, and usually we do this at the expense of the patient's comfort—his physical, financial, and emotional comfort.

The time has come for a new concept of prevention. It is not enough to find disease early or try to treat it more effectively—we must eradicate these notions. Once we find the problem, it is already too late. Real prevention means just that— do not let the problem occur. In this new scheme the patient is no longer a victim but an active participant in his own health. In fact, it is the person who creates his health. This involves reflection of life-style, on whether he thinks, acts, and eats in a way that is more natural. If not, he should not expect to be well and needs to change in order to improve. If his health is based on physical examinations and blood tests, he feels lucky and then walks on eggshells hoping his luck holds out. When a person actively creates his own health, he need not consider himself lucky. He had a lot to do with it and he knows why.

The answers to our problems cannot be imposed on us from without. Each person must look within, acknowledge the problem, then find an appropriate way out. But even though each individual must find his or her own way, we should all realize that any real solution cannot be a temporary one, for these we can no longer tolerate. We can no longer live day to day hoping that someone else will give us bread. It is time to start growing our own.

Diet, Behavior, and Rehabilitation

Frank Kern

Many years ago Dostoevski made a very sage and visionary statement. He said, "The degree of civilization in a society can be judged by entering its prisons."

According to this thinking, we are a truly sick and uncivilized world society. Today's statistics in the areas of crime and mental illness mirror the failure of the human service organizations in the United States and throughout the world.

The current numerical indictment includes over 12 million arrests of children for delinquent acts each year. Of these, more than 2,500,000 are formalized in the courts and criminal justice network. It might also be added that 85 percent of adult offenders were part of the juvenile justice system while growing up.

Alex Schauss, in his book *Diet, Crime and Delinquency*, estimates that, "At least one-and-a-half-million children will be the victims of parental abuse and neglect in 1980. Alcoholism cost the United States in 1978 over 8 billion dollars in lost revenues due to automobile accidents and acts of violence. On any given day in 1980, it is estimated that over one million people will be on probation or parole, while over 300,000 adult offenders await release from U.S. prisons. Estimates of the cost of maintaining the criminal justice system range from 30 to 50 billion dollars per year. Add to this total the monetary damage caused by criminals and estimates approach 200 billion dollars per year . . . . Environmental exposure to toxic metal lead has mushroomed to over 500 times that experienced by sixteenth century man. In 1971, the United States had the dubious distinction of becoming the first nation on earth to consume processed foods for more than 50 percent of its diet. Over 4,000 additives can now be found in the American food supply, none of which have ever been tested thoroughly for their effects on the central nervous system. We have become a nation of coffee and soda pop drinkers, fast food consumers, and refined carbohydrate junkies, without regard to their disastrous consequences, particularly on our children. Less than thirty-five years ago hyperactive children were a rarity. The incidence of hyperactivity and learning disability is higher in the United States than in any other country in the world!"

Coupled with this disheartening reality of crime in America, Richard C. Wertz, Chairman of the National Conference of State Criminal Justice Planning Administrators, testified before a U.S. Senate Subcommittee on State, Justice, Commerce, and the Judiciary in March of 1979 and stated: "Recent public opinion polls clearly indicate that the American people are fed-up with the violence and property loss caused in every community in the country by our lawless elements. They are fed-up with the inability of our police, courts, corrections and juvenile justice agencies to adequately deal with the criminal offender. No other domestic issue . . . not health care, not the energy problem, not even inflation . . . is of greater concern to more of our citizens."

The correctional and mental health systems are the only industries that succeed by their failures. Our prison and mental health populations grow larger not only because crime and mental illness are increasing, but also, because the people in these institutions often come out worse, commit more crimes, return to prisons and institutions, and continue through the revolving door of social rehabilitation in an endless cycle of crime, institution, crime, institution. This is because the objective of the criminal justice system is actually punishment, not rehabilitation.

In most states, 90 percent or more of prison expenditures go for custodial care in the form of guards, facilities, and new-wave prison technology. What is leftover goes for counseling, job training, and education.

The contributing factors to crime, delinquency, and antisocial behavior can be limitless. It is unfortunate that the "medical model" portrait of crime and behavior still revolves around the concepts of socio-economics, family birth ranking, fixations, toilet training—an entire spectrum of psychological factors. Dr. William H. Lyle, Jr., former Chief Psychologist for the Federal Bureau of Prisons, observes, "The courts' limited familiarity with these issues is compounded by the fact that psychologists and psychiatrists tend to reject metabolic, in preference to psychodynamic explanations, more out of ignorance of metabolic issues, unfortunately, than of awareness of them." Fortunately, the back to this attitude regarding behavior is that the conscientiousness of researchers is leading them into new arenas for answers. Contemporary research is now unearthing pragmatic alternatives.

Obviously, there has to be a better way, and there is. We have come to find out that sometimes the best solution is the most obscure or the most simple. The importance of diet and nutrition in any rehabilitation, whether it be of sickness and disease or antisocial behavior and crime is of paramount importance, especially when we understand just who commits crimes. Three out of four persons arrested for previous offenses are under twenty-five years of age and most of these are under twenty-one. This statistic alone verifies that much of the so-called crime wave is the result of the post-war baby boom, a bulging of the social age group most prone to violence and deviant behavior. When we couple this with the fact that at that time technological changes and perversions in the American food supply came about, it is no small wonder that devitalized food and disastrous amounts of sugar are causal effects of unacceptable behavior.[5]

---

[5] The relationship between sugar consumption and asocial behavior was evaluated in March, 1981 by Frank Kern and associates at the Tidewater Detention Home in Virginia. Commenting on the program in a letter to Mr. Kern, Stephen Schoenthaler, of the University of Southern Mississippi, stated:

"When you requested that my associates and I revise your institutional diet and measure the impact the change would have upon the incarcerated juveniles, I admit I was somewhat skeptical. Many theoretically sound programs in corrections have failed when carefully evaluated. Nevertheless, as an objective social scientist, I attempted to develop a valid unbiased research design which would be capable of measuring the impact of the dietary change. I have had the research design reviewed by several of my colleagues at Virginia Wesleyan College as well as peers in colleges and universities in Florida, Mississippi, South ▶

It is in this context that we must become aware of the direct cause and effect of food and nutrition on the rehabilitative process. The events of the present are crucial. Dietary patterns and the quality of food can affect, improve, and cure not only physical maladies, but mental and criminal manifestations as well. The brain is the most chemically sensitive organ in the body. The fact that our food supply is over-chemicalized seems to point to a direction that desperately needs to be investigated. Without first grounding our nervous systems through whole foods, the entire rehabilitative process at best will be mediocre.

It is our contention that with whole foods—and in particular the macrobiotic diet—we will establish new and creative methods for true rehabilitation.

Michio and Aveline Kushi, William Dufty, the entire network of macrobiotic teachers at the Kushi Institute and the East West Centers throughout the United States and the world, are undoubtedly at the vanguard of true holistic health care and social rehabilitation.

They are the social messengers of our time regarding the entire plane of healing, health care, and individual growth and development. Please heed their message of a natural, traditional philosophy of food, health, existence, and social harmony.

▶Carolina, and Louisiana. There is a consensus that the design is not flawed.

"As you recall, the primary goal was to modify the children's diet in such a manner that it would be (1) politically noncontroversial by being consistent with accepted medical standards, (2) financially practical, (3) easy to implement in other institutions, and (4) capable of being scientifically evaluated. Using these guidelines, a simple reduction in sucrose seemed to be the best initial project. The literature on sugar strongly suggests that a reduction in sugar consumption has no adverse effects and is associated with the elimination or reduction of several negative behavioral characteristics such as hypertension, violent behavior, and delinquency.

"The results of the study are truly amazing. The incidence of misbehavior resulting in institutional discipline has dropped 45 percent. It is important to state that the success of the project depended upon keeping the nine staff members who ultimately made the decisions to formally discipline the children unaware of the research. If they knew that the project was being done, they might have become more lenient and thereby made the project invalid. Therefore, keeping the staff in a state of ignorance was absolutely necessary.

"Statistically, the likelihood of the results having been due to random variation in the juvenile population is less than one percent. In short, the reduction of sugar consumption by the children seems to have almost cut the incidence of infractions in half. Neither my colleagues nor myself have been able to create an alternative explanation for this phenomenal success."

New Dimensions in Nursing

Kristen Schmidt, R.N.

It is common knowledge that there is an upheaval in nursing today. In February of 1981, the American Hospital Association held a national investigation which revealed that nurses are leaving the profession because of economic, political, educational, and status deficits. However, I would like to suggest that the underlying reason is much deeper; nurses have lost their dream. To me, a dream has something to do with aesthetics and intangibles; not so much with material acquisitions or prestige. I will share with you my own dream upon entering nursing school, and in so doing reflect on what other nurses' aspirations are as well.

I had hoped to achieve a sense of personal growth, worth, and actualization. I wanted to have intimate contact with people and effect a change in their lives. I wanted to contribute something valuable to society, and to strengthen and work with people's support system. In becoming a nurse, I hoped to be able to directly influence a person's health. Working with the patient and family would be working with a mini-society. But most exciting and challenging was the idea that there is a creative art to the profession of care for people.

The Traditional Nurse

Nursing has always been in existence; it is not necessary to go to school to become a nurse. In America, the profession of nursing began when the Civil War demanded the need for an organization of women to care for the sick and wounded. After the war, "centers of hospitality" arose, but often the nurse went to the home. In the course of aiding in a patient's recovery, the nurse had a wide range of responsibilities. She provided personal care by bathing, grooming, massaging and exercising the patient. Medically, the nurse prepared and administered herbal medications, applied external plasters, fomentations and compresses. She was an acute observer of her patient's emotions, behavior, and response to physical stimuli. In care of the patient's surroundings, she brightened or darkened the "sick room" depending upon his or her need. The room was kept clean and orderly. A soothing emotional environment was provided to induce relaxation which enhanced the healing process. Part of her day was spent reading and conversing with her patient.

The nurse was a liaison between the patient and family. Information was gathered from the family to aid in her assessment and plan of care. Frequent reports of the patient's changing condition were mediated by the nurse. Since she was closest to the patient during his illness, she did collaborative work with the physician. He depended on her observations and intuition to make his diagnosis and formulate a treatment plan.

Education of the patient and family was another responsibility. In simple terms, she explained how to restore and maintain health.

Perhaps the nurse's most sagacious and powerful role was that of moral counselor. She understood that along with sickness comes regression, depression, and dependency. Having nothing to do and nowhere to go, the patient would often re-examine the priorities in his life. Her counsel and assistance for the patient's self-reflection were always available. The old schools of nursing taught that the nurse should be cheerful and optimistic. She was the patient's biggest advocate. Her intention for a good recovery set the tone for everything she did with her patient. She was an inspiration to his confidence, providing constant encouragement and support. Above all, she understood that personality and behavior were not independent of scientific knowledge and medicine.

Traditional and Macrobiotic Nursing

What the nurse used to do made her function valuable and gave her a sense of autonomy because she saw a direct improvement from her interactions with the patient. She was realizing her dream. Nurses today spend more time interacting with machines than patients; as a result, they are not directly responsible for positive results. Their self worth is challenged.

The traditional nurse and macrobiotic nurse are consorts. They both show an awareness as to whether a patient's overall energy is functioning properly. During the course of daily patient care this can be accomplished in various ways:

1. Touch

Energy runs through twelve pathways (meridians) in the body. Touch subtly but powerfully affects the quality of energy flowing through the meridians.[6] The traditional nurse was well educated in the technique and importance of massage, bathing, external applications and general personal care of her patient. Her touch was an art, highly regarded by the patient. Macrobiotics teaches *shiatsu* (pressure point massage) and acupuncture. Both are used to stimulate and release energy, as diagnostic tools, as methods of analgesia and anesthesia, and in the treatment of illness.

2. Nutrition

The old school recognized the importance of high quality, well balanced and properly cooked food, both as a vehicle to recovery and as an intergral part of the maintenance of good health. Macrobiotics teaches that foods such as whole grains, beans, and vegetables, which were the traditional foods of our ancestors, provide the optimum balance of all the necessary nutrients to enhance a healthy body, keeping the mind and body clear for the free flow of energy.

3. Emotional Interaction

The traditional and macrobiotic nurse both help the patient express his concerns and feelings. Talking, crying, laughing, and singing are extractions of emotional energy. Verbal interchange transfers energy between the patient and nurse. Often,

---

[6] Please refer to the *Book of Dō-In: Exercise for Physical and Spiritual Development* by Michio Kushi (Japan Publications, Inc.) for a discussion of the energy meridians which have been used for thousands of years in the practice of acupuncture, *shiatsu*, *Dō-In* (self-massage) and other traditional Oriental therapies.

the patient will feel relaxed and relieved after a good conversation. Compassion and the intent of wellness are in a sense high quality "emotional food" offered by the nurse to her patient.

4. Observation

Before the advent of machinery as a tool for charting and observation, the nurse of yesteryear relied on her six senses (sight, sound, touch, hearing, taste, perception) as tools for monitoring her patient's changing condition. This was a well developed art and science. Observations of body flexibility and tension, pain threshold, skin color, texture, and temperature, bodily smell, the patient's voice and body sounds (i.e., bowel peristalisis, rales in lungs), and behavioral patterns were all important factors in this process. She had an understanding that the external manifestation of signs and symptoms reflected the internal condition of the body.

The macrobiotic methods of diagnosis are easily integrated in this process.[7] Certain areas of the face and body relate directly to organs and systems (digestive, reproductive, respiratory, circulatory, nervous, endocrine). With these methods, a nurse can immediately understand the patient's condition before the manifestation of physical signs and symptoms. This method can be valuable because it does not have the danger of side effects, nor the expense of extensive technological testing.

Studies

What are some of the tangible effects of these methods in the restoration of a patient's health today?

1. Touch

Delores Krieger, R.N., Ph.D. (Professor of Nursing, New York University) began her practice and research into therapeutic touch in 1969. She theorizes that there is a transfer of energy from healer to patient that is "done physiologically by a kind of electron transfer resonance."[8] At the Langly Porter Neuropsychiatric Institute, U.C.L.A., San Francisco, her methodology was tested with highly sophisticated equipment. "Mr. A. . . . had had severe neck and back pain for several years following the injection of contrast dye into the spinal canal for myographic studies. Since then, he had been unable to walk down a flight of stairs without the aid of crutches." After therapeutic touch, "Mr. A. walked out of the laboratory, down a standard flight of stairs, and out to the street carrying his crutches . . ."[9] A woman with fibroid tumors, upon follow-up examination after therapeutic touch, had no tumors to be found in her uterus. In another case, the severity of chronic migraine headaches in a young woman was diminished.

Ms. Krieger's technique is being taught as a part of the Master's Program in nursing at New York University and is presented in universities and hospitals

---

[7] Please refer to *How to See Your Health: The Book of Oriental Diagnosis* by Michio Kushi (Japan Publications, Inc.) for a discussion of these traditional methods.

[8] Kreiger, Delores, R.N., Ph.D. "Therapeutic Touch: Searching for Evidence of Philosophical Change." American Journal of Nursing, April 1979, pp. 660–62.

[9] Ibid.

throughout the United States. Other nurses have followed Ms. Krieger's path and found this method of vibrational healing to be beneficial in the patients they treat.[10]

2. Nutrition

Michio Kushi has found that the quality of food can be directly responsible for the cause, and in many instances, the relief of most degenerative diseases. Whole grains, vegetables, beans, and other natural, traditional foods contain the highest quality nutritional energy. When cooked properly and eaten on a daily basis, more balanced foods can heal the body naturally and completely. The case histories in this volume offer examples of this.

3. Emotion

Norman Cousins' initial diagnosis was progressive paralysis. He arrested and improved this degenerative collogen disease by laughing. He discovered that depression impairs the body's immunological function, and that positive emotions produce positive chemical changes.[11]

O. Carl Simonton, M.D., Stephanie Matthews-Simonton, and James Creighton have spent years researching the positive effects of visualization on the eradication of cancer as a supplement to orthodox medical treatment. Their clinical findings show that through the patient's self-expression of wellness (utilizing physical exercise, imagery, and art), cancer can be arrested and reversed.[12]

The physical environment seems to make a difference in the recovery rate of hospitalized patients. Studies suggest that the artificiality of intensive care units, with their noisy equipment, florescent lights, intravenous feeding and the unfamiliar faces of the medical team, traumatize the already sick person and could further impair his or her healing ability.

The Dilemma in Nursing

The dilemma facing nurses today is that many have allowed themselves to believe that pushing a button will give them a sense of professional satisfaction and self-worth. The problem is not technology itself, but the abuse of it.

If the nurse's dream is to relate to people, it goes unrealized because she is limited by the scope of machines. If her dream is to be a liaison between the patient and family, she is left in a relationship with a machine. Technology and the hospital demand that the nurse be an expert mechanic and druggist. She finds herself apathetic and exhausted with frustration. Eventually, she may quit the profession completely.

Macrobiotic health care does not foster this dependency. Through the use of palm healing, *shiatsu*, diet, and compassion, the macrobiotic nurse resumes the role of her older sister, the traditional nurse. She realizes her dream.

---

[10] Quin, Janet F., R.N., M.A. "One Nurse's Evolution as a Healer." American Journal of Nursing, April 1979, pp. 662–64.

[11] Macrae, Janet, R.N., M.A., "Therapeutic Touch in Illness." American Journal of Nursing, April 1979, pp. 664–65, Cousins, Norman. *The Anatomy of an Illness*, W.W. Norton & Co., 1979.

[12] Simonton, Carl O., Matthews-Simonton, Stephanie, Creighton, James. *Getting Well Again*, Los Angeles: J.P. Tarcher, Inc., 1978.

Prevention as a Social Priority

William Tara

In talking of prevention we not only have to talk about food, but also about some other very important social issues and the way in which they are related to our diet and the way that we live our lives.

All of the statistical data point to the fact that there is not one of us who is really healthy. When we take into account the incidences of nervous diseases, mental illness, cancer, heart disease, diabetes, multiple sclerosis, and so forth, it turns out that more than 100 percent of the population is affected. This is a pretty frightening situation, one that demands our full attention in forming social priorities.

The connection between diet, heart disease, cancer, and other ailments has been known for some time. Research was begun in this area as early as 1919, and very profound statistical correlations were made between different types of heart disease, cancer, and food patterns.

In 1977, *Dietary Goals for the United States* was released by the Senate Select Committee on Nutrition and Human Needs. Unfortunately, however, the news that food might be responsible for many of the problems that we are facing was on page one for a day, page two for two days—and then it disappeared.

There was no government action after that, no great change in medical attitudes and, more importantly, no significant change in public attitudes. The roots of this problem do not lie within the food industry nor within medical institutions; they lie within the population of the country and within the basic attitudes we have about health and our ability to change our own health.

One attitude that must change is that of responsibility. This word is often used today and it has become quite fashionable to talk about taking responsibility for one's health or for one's life, but responsibility is a double edged sword. In order to be really responsible, we must have the ability to respond. Responsibility is not an intellectual concept but rather a projection of our own sensitivity. And our irresponsibility in dealing with our own health is something that has been ingrained in us from the earliest possible age.

We can do something about this in school children, and in our education of the young, by teaching them to have tools available so that they can do something about that responsibility. But it is very difficult for those of us who are adults because we have to go through a de-education process.

In my own practice of macrobiotics over the past fifteen years, I have been in several situations in which problems have come up concerning my own health and the health of my children. And instantaneously, from somewhere deep in my consciousness, comes the reaction, "Go to the doctor!" It may be a situation that is not so serious. In fact, it may be quite simple, but the depth of our own conditioning brings forth that response. One time, my daughter had a fever when she was about five months old. The fever went up and then it dropped. I thought everything was all right but then twenty-four hours later it rose again and I panicked. I called up a friend of mine who had several children and said that I did not know what to do about it. "Is she cutting teeth?" my friend asked. When I said yes, I was told that that was the reason; that a fever often comes when children are cutting teeth. I had not known that. My own education was incomplete concerning children and the types of changes that are normal when they are growing up. And so I immediately contacted someone who knew better than I. Nowadays, however, we increasingly cut ourselves off from traditional information sources. For instance, we often cut oursleves off from our parents, grandparents, and other family members who have the experience of living. We have devalued the experience of living. We have to reinstitute that process.

Another problem which interferes with our developing good preventive programs is the frequently patronizing attitude of the medical community as a whole when it comes to relating information to the layperson. When information is given to those of us who are not a part of the medical community, it is often mystified. The language is not commonly known. Information is often left out that is crucial to our understanding. This is especially true when we are dealing with information concerning prevention.

Perhaps their point of view is that the average person cannot possibly understand what goes on in his or her body. But if we cannot understand, who can? We may not understand it at the level of someone who had studied anatomy and physiology for many years, but we can understand the basic life processes which are not, however, taught to us in school. Especially basic processes like daily nutrition. I have talked to doctors who have said that in all their years of medical training they had about six or seven hours of lectures on nutrition and its importance. Then we wonder why there are problems with the kind of health care there is in society. We are not directing ourselves to health at all, we are directing ourselves to sickness. In the Western world, to my awareness, we have no health services at all, only sickness services.

A health service implies that the priority of the service is to create health, and not to try to alleviate the symptoms of illness after they have occurred. At present, the priority of preventive programs within government and the medical profession is extremely low. In some cases it involves less than 1 percent of the total expenditure of money.

With all due respect to the many conscientious people in the research field, I do not feel it is necessary to wait until all of the information is in before we act. If there is a reasonable suspicion that something we are doing in our daily life is detrimental to our health and well-being, and that of the next generation, we should automatically take steps to curtail that. Not through legislation but through education.

In many cases the preventive aspects of disease are already known to a great extent. The National Cancer Institute has stated that food may be a more prevalent factor than tobacco in the development of cancer. And yet one never sees a warning on the side of a food package from the Surgeon General stating that consuming this is detrimental to health and can cause cancer. Why is it not on there? Could it be that commercial interests are too great in that area? Could it be that we have not really developed a commitment within ourselves to make those kind of changes, that it is easier to pick out one factor which is simple to target and concentrate on and let all the rest slide?

A proper attitude toward health must come from each of us. If it does not come from the population in general, it will not come from up high on the pyramid. Because there is no pressure from the public, people can stay in laboratories for years and do detailed studies which yield little in the way of practical application. For example, if it is discovered that one particular fatty acid is more detrimental than another, the next step is often to try to find out what it is inside that fatty acid which is causing the problem. This detailed information can be useful if we funnel it back through society and use it as a course to take action. Otherwise it is a waste of time and money, and we cannot afford to waste either in the present situation that we are in.

Another thing about which we have to be very clear when we talk about prevention is the false hope syndrome which frequently comes out of modern medicine. In Europe now, not a week goes by when you do not read something in the newspaper about Interferon in cancer research. Interferon is a substance which occurs naturally in the body and which in some laboratory tests inhibits cancer growth or the growth of cancer cells. It is being used experimentally and costs about $50,000 a treatment. Tremendous effort is going into the research of this drug. I have had people with cancer come to the Community Health Foundation in London, and ask, "Should I change my daily diet or should I hold out and see what happens with Interferon?" This is because it is said that we are right on the brink of a breakthrough. But how many times in the last fifteen years have we heard that we are on the brink of a breakthrough?

I do not feel that we need any more proof about the connection between diet, life-style, and disease. I think that it is absolutely necessary that research and laboratory work go on, but I think that we also need to break out of this cocoon of impotence and start to look at and value the experiences of our fellow human beings. We have brains, we can make value judgments. If we see a situation in which someone has made a simple change in their life and profound changes have resulted, we need to examine that. We must decide whether we need to start applying that experience to our own lives or experimenting on our own. We have become too frightened to experiment. We have to put a little bit of adventure back in life again. Not false adventure, nor the vicarious adventures of television and movies, but the real adventure of living.

There is an ancient Chinese greeting that goes, "May you live in difficult times." If you live in difficult times you have the greatest potential to realize your own self. When you come up against difficulties you can grow, you can develop. We do live in difficult times but we are only fortunate if we can grasp the opportunity to demonstrate that we are up to the challenges. Those challenges do not depend on any select portion of the population, they depend upon all of us equally. I hope that we are up to the challenge. I think that we are.

Lemuel Shattuck Hospital Macrobiotic Food Program

Introduction

The macrobiotic food program at the Lemuel Shattuck Hospital in Jamaica Plain, Massachusetts is a daily meals program that has served the staff of the hospital since March, 1980. It entered its second intended phase as a patient meal program for elderly mental patients in February, 1982, under the supervision of Dr. Jonathan Lieff, Chief of Psychiatry.

The Shattuck program has thus far resulted in a substantial acceptance by hospital staff. It is anticipated to yield positive results in the overall physical and mental conditions of the elderly patients who are scheduled to be enrolled. The development of an effective and flexible patient meal system on this small initial scale will make possible the assignment of other patients in other wards of the Shattuck Hospital to such an alternative diet.

History

In August of 1980 we first met with the current Director of the Shattuck Hospital, Paul Schulman, through an introduction by Dr. Lieff. Mr. Schulman expressed his and the administration's interest in beginning an alternative food program in the cafeteria. This would be the first step toward the practical development of patient meal programs as part of a general "wellness" program. It was felt that in this way the staff could develop an awareness and support of the basic concept of patient meals, and in addition, also benefit from the meals. We were subsequently invited to become members of the dietary department for the planning of this first phase, which was completed by the end of November with the helpful advice of Thomas J. Kelly, Director of Food Service.

At about this time Mr. Schulman decided to leave the Shattuck Hospital for work in the private sector. However, the hiring of an additional full-time macrobiotic crew of five was completed before his departure.

There was some delay in initiating the necessary food purchases due to the newness of many of the items within the structure of the state purchasing system. During this time, we met with the new Director, Mr. William Goyette, who was willing to go ahead with the program. He outlined his criteria for success over a two-month trial period: that food costs be comparable to the cost of regular meals and that there be general acceptance of the meals by the staff.

The staff meal program—a lunchtime meal Mondays through Fridays—was begun on March 9, 1980 and has fulfilled these criteria.

In the beginning, meals were served from separate lines to allow the choice of a full macrobiotic meal or a full regular meal. During this separate serving period of two months, food quantities and costs were recorded in detail and the average and total costs computed regularly. The average cost per meal was between $1.15 and 59 cents per meal; cost variations being mainly attributable to ingredients used (e.g., fish as opposed to all-vegetarian) and the total number of meals served (the cost per meal declining with an increase in the total number served).

In addition, overall staff response has been favorable; in our estimation, the cafeteria patronage has nearly doubled for the noontime meal, and (since the integration of the two serving lines allows arbitrary choice) approximately 70 to 85 percent of all meals served have at least one macrobiotic menu item in them by customer request, with requests for additional items and full macrobiotic meals (currently about 35 percent) increasing steadily as customers become familiar with our products on a daily basis. Ongoing favorable comments reflect an appreciation for the interesting, flavorful, and attractively prepared food found in the macrobiotic menu and the fresh experience for many staff members of being exposed to a very personal educational opportunity in the form of food.

Since the last precise tabulation of meal costs quoted above, daily menus have been developed utilizing progressively less expensive ingredients (including USDA surplus grains, beans, etc.) with a continued success in acceptance and appreciation of the taste and health qualities of macrobiotic food by the hospital staff. Our most recent cost estimates show that, with frequent inclusion of fish, menus can be prepared at an average cost of 61 cents per meal over a two-week period, with costs as low as 38 cents per meal.

Current Status and Future Implications

The preparation and serving of food to the initial group of twenty-eight elderly mental patients will, we feel, accomplish three objectives: 1) a rapid transition for a relatively stable patient population to an unprecedented daily diet of primarily vegetable-quality whole foods (and the concurrent fulfillment of RDA's with such a diet through cooperation with hospital dietitians); 2) the implementation of a workable "food delivery" system—from preparation to patient feeding—within the existing structure of the institution; and 3) the relief of many stress and nutritional symptoms now experienced by these patients, reducing or eliminating the need for ongoing medication and/or restraint. This final aspect will be under formal study by Dr. Lieff's staff during the course of one year.

The relative familiarity of the hospital as a whole with macrobiotic food will be, we feel, the most important factor in the success of the patient program. The fact that the macrobiotic food program has survived three changes in administration at the Shattuck is a fair testament to its general acceptance.

The program as a whole, for both staff and patients, is approaching the phase of being a manageable routine—able to be duplicated in any institution of like size—for the delivery of alternative diet. We look forward, when this stage is completed, to creating further opportunities for effective health care through the implementation of educational programs, volunteer and intern services in supplemental traditional therapies, and the encouragement of accompanying research by participating health professionals.

Thomas J. Iglehart
Eric Zutrau
February, 1982

Chapter 5

Case Histories

Cancer and Cancer Related

Choriocarcinoma

John Jodziewicz
Allentown, Pennsylvania

On Friday, March 17, 1980, I was laid off from my job at a stove factory in a small rural town in northeast Pennsylvania. I was twenty-three years old, engaged to be married, and a recent college graduate. My plans for the future were to go on to study cultural and physical geography at a graduate school, but I was not absolutely sure; I was feeling somewhat aimless.

The following Monday, I went to see a doctor about the swelling and hardness of my left testicle. In 1977 I had first noticed a pea-sized hardness there. During the winter of 1979–1980 it increased in size, while a lump appeared on my neck. "It's probably a hydrocele, and the doctor will just drain it," I told Ingrid, my fiancee, "and the lump in my neck is just from all these fevers I've been having."

As soon as the doctor saw me, he had me admitted to Allentown Sacred Heart Hospital for a radical orchiectomy, which means they removed my left testicle. They then told me that I had a very advanced (fourth stage) case of pure chorio-carcinoma. I vividly remember sitting in the hospital room, with Ingrid at my side, listening to two oncologists and a resident physician tell us that I had a "one-percent chance to live out the year, even with chemotherapy." Also, the disease had spread to my left kidney, both lungs, and neck.

It was hard for me to believe that I had terminal cancer. To me, this was as traumatic as when my mother died of diabetes in 1971. I was sure that my "any-thing but meat" diet, megadoses of vitamins and supplements, and rugged outdoor activities protected me from disease. But here Ingrid and I sat, being told that I would most probably die before my twenty-fourth birthday.

During the next four months I had fevers, nosebleeds, constipation, difficulty breathing, a persistent cough, skin discoloration, total hair loss, chills, loss of appetite, headaches, fatigue, severe mouth ulcers, nausea, vomiting, bone marrow depression, dizziness, total body arthritic pain, hypersensitivity of the scalp, ringing in the ears, and loosening teeth. This was the most horrible time in my life; and these symptoms were not as a result of the cancer, but of the treatment called chemotherapy. These courses of chemical "therapy" included being attached, intravenously, to an IVAC machine for 168 hours (seven days), going home for two weeks (and being very ill), then coming back in for another 168 hours.

After two cycles of treatment, the doctors told me that there was no significant change in the size of my many tumors. They would check the sizes through x-rays and by measuring the size of the lump on my neck, which, they said, corresponded to all the other tumors. My doctors conferred with an internationally respected specialist of testicular cancer, who advised experimental dosages of drugs. I was told by one of my oncologists that they had never given such high doses of drugs to anyone under their care before. He warned that the dosages could kill me. He also told Ingrid and me that if the tumors remained after two more cycles of treatment, I would die in two months (August, 1980).

The first cycle was administered. The tumors remained. During the second, and last, cycle of chemotherapy (end of May), my stepmother, father, and Ingrid held me as I wretched and convulsed. I felt that death was near. The next night a priest gave me rites. After the treatment was done the tumors remained. My three oncologists made three different remarks to me: "There's not much more we can do," one said as he looked at his papers; "You always have a 50–50 chance in everything," said another as he looked out toward the mountains through my window; "You'll have a couple of months," said the third, as he stared at the floor. They wanted to test my lungs and kidneys for possible damage due to the chemotherapy.

Two things that would change my life had happened, one before my last course of chemotherapy, and another during the treatment. Just before my last "bout with chemo," I was introduced to Denny Waxman, former director of the East West Foundation in Philadelphia, by a good friend named Kurt Maute. Denny explained the macrobiotic approach. It was interesting, but I was not convinced it would help me. The diet he recommended was comprised of about 50 percent whole cereal grains, 30 percent locally grown vegetables, 10 percent beans and sea vegetables, 5 percent *misp* soup, and 5 percent condiments. I kept his advice in the back of my mind.

The other experience was of a spiritual nature. While I was at the hospital my deceased mother told me in a dream that I should go to Montreal and crawl up the steps of Saint Joseph's Oratory in prayer. So, I decided to try the macrobiotic diet and to go to Montreal.

As I went up the hillside on my knees I was in a trance, as if I blended into the mountain the church sat upon. All of a sudden I felt peaceful, and positive that if I changed my way of life and ate macrobiotically, I would get better.

During the end of June, 1980, I met Michio Kushi, who gave me advice about how to get better. He said that I should follow the diet and seek guidance from macrobiotic teachers. Ingrid and I both felt that this was more than a diet, that it was a way of life based on the natural laws of the universe. Three times a week we would drive 70 miles to Philadelphia to study cooking, learn more about macrobiotics, and make new friends. I read every book I could get my hands on about macrobiotics. In two weeks all pain went away; in two months the tumor in my neck shrunk to half its previous size. Here it was, August, and I felt strong and getting stronger. One day I went hiking in the mountains and my dog could not keep up with me.

Ingrid was my cook, my inspiration, and my love. She suffered and sacrificed so much for me. But ultimately it was my responsibility; I was the one who had made myself sick, so I would make myself well. By May, 1981 I felt so well that I asked Dr. Richard Donze, a good friend who is also macrobiotic, if he could have a blood test done on me. Results showed no cancer.

It has been twenty-one months now since I was supposed to have died. I think there are five reasons why I am, instead, so well and healthy. They are: 1) total support from family and friends; 2) correct macrobiotic practice, no binging; 3) a strong natural immune system; 4) gratitude for all dfficulties, for they help me to develop; and to God, the Infinite; and 5) the will to get better. I am not only physically healthy, but I feel spiritually healthy as well. This clean, natural diet and way of life has enhanced and broadened my perspective of the Catholic tradition in which I was raised.

Ingrid and I plan to study and teach macrobiotics for the rest of our lives, have a large family, and write a book on our "adventure." We also envision our children inheriting a healthy and peaceful world.

Granular Myoblastoma on the Vocal Cord

Laura Ann Fitzpatrick
Sherborn, Massachussetts
(With Mrs. Phyllis Fitzpatrick)

Laura: It was in the spring of 1979 that I was diagnosed as having a tumor on the vocal cords after my voice was getting raspy. I had tried out for cheerleading at my high school and had to tell my friends to be patient because I could not use my voice. That summer, in August, I had an operation on my throat in which the tumor was removed.

Mrs. Fitzpatrick: Laura's voice had completely left her. I simply felt she had been using her voice too much. We finally took her to the doctor who discovered a node on her vocal cords, recommending that she have an operation. A tumor was found, and we had to wait a few days to discover whether or not it was malignant. It turned out to be granular myoblastoma, a rare type of benign tumor. In fact, Laura's case was the only one where the tumor was on the vocal cord.

In January, 1980, we went to see a surgeon at Boston's University Hospital who specialized in laser beam surgery. It was discovered that the tumor had definitely returned following its removal in August. After the second operation, the doctor was quite sure that the laser surgery was successful and that the tumor was gone.

However, Laura's voice temporarily left her after the second operation, and during the four-week checkup following surgery, the doctor was not pleased with what he saw, since the tumor seemed to be returning. He did not want to discourage us completely, but he said that there was definite swelling. He advised Laura to return every three months for close monitoring.

In February, 1980, we saw a television program featuring Professor Jean Kohler describing his recovery from pancreatic cancer through macrobiotics. At that time we signed up for a three-day *Cancer and Diet* seminar offered through the East West Foundation. At first, my husband John and I felt uncomfortable because we saw many people who seemed to be very ill. When Michio Kushi entered, however, a comfort and calm came over me, and I began to feel very much at home. Mr. Kushi opened the seminar with a warm welcome and said "How many people

here have cancer?" Among the young and old people in the room, half of the
hands were raised. I was impressed by his relaxed and sensible approach, and the
simplicity of his presentation. At the end of those three days, I tried to digest all
of my notes. Laura, who had not attended the workshop, felt the excitement that
John and I felt about the information gained during the weekend.

We called Michio Kushi to make an appointment. He told Laura that this would
be very simple—to not be at all discouraged. He could support her recovery by
recommending "a very simple diet."

Laura: We began to introduce this way of eating to our family, and with two
sisters and three brothers still at home, this became quite an adventure. We
cleaned out the cupboards and moved the remaining food to another section. I
just loved the food. We invited an experienced macrobiotic cook to come into
our home to prepare the food, and it was delicious to me from the very beginning.
My eleven-year-old brother's first question was "What do you do on birthdays?"
He knew that this would be a change, but he was concerned that the change
would be forever, and that he would no longer enjoy his meals. My sisters immediately went on the diet.

Mrs. Fitzpatrick: John and I both wanted to support Laura, and we also began
to eat in this new way as much as we could. We changed our stove from electric to
gas, and the adventures continued as we truly tried to understand the principles
behind the diet. Laura temporarily went on a more restricted diet which did not
include oil. She also went to bed with taro potato plasters wrapped around her
neck.

Laura: I experienced many changes throughout my body because toxins were
being released rapidly. As a result I felt a great deal more energy, though my voice
was still raspy and weak. I was going to a special therapist who was teaching me
to express myself despite the weakness of my voice.

As I continued with the diet, however, my voice definitely started improving,
becoming less raspy. We were noticing changes that were taking place, but were
concentrating on the diet rather than the tumor.

In early spring, when we met with the doctor, I was shocked to find that no
operation was necessary. There was still scar tissue from the first operation but
my condition was greatly improved. The doctor suggested that we check on my
condition every three months.

Mrs. Fitzpatrick: Laura's condition continued to improve through the fall.
Every three months she returned to the doctor who found that her condition
remained stable. There was no suggestion of further surgery.

Laura: In November, I started to deviate from the recommended diet. I began
cooking with oil, ate turkey at Thanksgiving, and continued in this way until
Christmas, 1980. Symptoms started to return during that time, for example, my
voice grew weak and continually got worse. We went back for a checkup with the
doctor, although I knew that I was the one who was controlling my situation or
pushing it out of control. When the doctor saw me, he said that the tumor was
again large and had to be operated on immediately. This was in January of 1981.
I cried and immediately understood what the problem was. At that point we asked

for a two-month reprieve. The doctor consented, saying that two months was not that crucial, especially after we explained that the diet had been helping my condition and that we understood what was happening. We immediately called Michio Kushi.

Mrs. Fitzpatrick: He looked at Laura and immediately saw that she had been cheating.

Laura: He scolded me humorously, and I decided I was ready to get back to basics and resume the diet he had recommended.

Mrs. Fitzpatrick: This experience brought home how difficult it was for Laura to practice the diet in the middle of her active life. Other people did not understand the situation. For example, college attendance is very difficult because dormitories and cafeterias tend not to encourage a more natural diet and way of life. Support of family and friends is such an important part of maintaining balance.

Laura: At this point, Michio recommended that I be even more careful with my diet for two months, so that my return to the doctor would be successful. I again began to discharge a lot of mucus and felt a tremendous cleansing coming very rapidly. I resumed the taro potato compresses each night. One humorous sidelight of this was that my father's T-shirts were disappearing, and he would find them with mysterious brown spots from the remains of the taro potato. I found that whenever I missed the ginger and taro potato plaster compress for a few days, the mucus would not discharge as freely. I prepared all the compresses by myself and the routine became normal. We maintained our sense of humor during this period, and the family would often joke about the daily events.

In March I spent two weeks as a guest at the Kushi house. Everyone in the house was so warm and helpful, and special breakfasts and lunches were prepared for me to eat during my school days. We returned to the doctor in June, following this two-month practice, and he was again surprised at the incredible progress I had made. I would see one of two doctors every three months, and they were maintaining contact with each other to monitor my progress. One is on the staff of the Leonard Morse Hospital, and the other is with the Boston University Hospital. The doctor at Leonard Morse saw that the tumor was in a very stable, improved condition, and that we again had nothing to worry about.

I learned from this experience that the diet makes sense. I know that it is my responsibility to maintain this way of life. I have learned a lot about myself and have gained a great deal of confidence from this experience.

Mrs. Fitzpatrick: I feel that Laura has grown considerably during this past year. I strongly believe that negative situations can create positive results, provided that attitude and practice work together. It is most important that a person facing a negative situation does not give up. Rather, it is important to open your eyes and gain confidence that something will come along that will work. We were very fortunate to have found this way of life before it became too late. If Laura had had more operations, her voice would have continued to grow worse. Macrobiotics gave her the opportunity to learn to take advantage of the many opportunities that are available to everyone who reaches out to accept the positive beginning.

Laura: I know how hard it may seem for someone to adopt this way of life because it is out of the ordinary. I stress, though, that it can be done. Macrobiotics works, if one has the desire to try.

Mrs. Fitzpatrick: As a family macrobiotics brought us much closer, because we all had one center of mutual interest in helping Laura to become well. We found unity and strength in sharing this important aspect of life.

Malignant Melanoma, Stage IV

Virginia Brown
Tunbridge, Vermont

On August 28, 1978, I was diagnosed by my doctor at the Burlington, Vermont Medical Center as having malignant melanoma in the fourth stage. Cancer was something I thought I never would have. At first it was so frightening knowing and feeling something alien in my body that I could not combat. This was very difficult for me, as I have too much pride to give in to anything.

The doctors wanted to remove the lymph glands and go from there, and they were very upset when I refused. Even though I had been trained and practiced in the medical profession for years, I could not go along. I had professed alternatives for years, but did not really practice them, so I believe, along with poor diet, frustration, and stress, that the cancer was given to me as a challenge.

I went to the East West Foundation Cancer Conference at Amherst in the summer of 1978, at the suggestion of my son and daughter-in-law, and was very impressed and started the Standard Macrobiotic Diet that same day. At the time I could hardly make it upstairs and was sleeping most of the day. I had no energy, no ambition, and my mind was dull and cloudy.

Within a week I noticed a drastic change in my energy level, attitude, and mental clarity.

I had an appointment with Mr. Kushi in September. I was told what to eat, how to cook, and to live a normal and active life. I also saw a Korean yoga teacher who put me on corrective and strengthening exercises. I also meditated and prayed.

I amazed myself at my perseverance, not one of my better qualities. Probably just stubbornness. My family all agreed with my decision and helped in all ways.

There have been all kinds of days—angry, crying, pain, weakness, tension, sadness, and hopelessness, but also thankful times. It has definitely been a challenge.

Reading everything I could about the macrobiotic way of life has been a great help. Through my experience, the most difficult thing has been to see other loved ones go the chemotherapy and radiation route and suffer so.

In October, 1979, Mr. Kushi said I was cured. I am continuing to eat and live macrobiotically, as I have far to go. I can also say that I am thankful for having had the disease, and to have experienced the wonder of the cure and the knowledge that we are what we eat and can change ourselves and the whole world.

In the Fall of 1979 I had the great pleasure of being able to take the Level I course at the Kushi Institute in Brookline and to work at the Erewhon warehouse.

The experience and people were wonderful and I am now inspired to share my knowledge with others.

My love and thanks to everyone.

Metastatic Prostate Cancer

Irving Malow
Evanston, Illinois
(Contributed by Keith Block, M.D.)

A sixty-year-old caucasian gentleman, Mr. Irving Malow, visited my office on September 24, 1980, virtually riddled with cancerous lesions on the spine, pelvis, and shoulders; secondary to his earlier diagnosis of prostate cancer. Mr. Malow experienced his initial symptoms and diagnosis in 1975. His disease process progressed from that time with a steady deterioration in his health. Prior conventional therapy included a partial orchiectomy, radiation therapy, and chemotherapy consisting of adriamycin, cytoxan, and cis-platinum. He stopped cytoxan and adriamycin after three treatments and stopped cis-platinum after one quarter of the treatment. During his regimen of cis-platinum chemotherapy, Mr. Malow threw up several times every hour for the following twelve hours until quitting the treatment. Further recommendations for chemotherapy were answered by Mr. Malow's firm statement: "I refuse to go on with these debilitating and torturous treatments."

During the time of his visit he expressed a definitive opinion refusing "under any circumstances" further chemotherapy (due to previous ill side-effects) other than the hormone stilbesterol. (*Note*: Mr. Malow had reduced his stilbesterol dosage by 50 percent just four weeks after initiation of the macrobiotic diet and reduced this still further to a quarter of his original dosage by his own volition from one-eighth to one-sixteenth of the original dosage and finally went off this medication completely.)

While practicing the prescribed macrobiotic dietary program, Mr. Malow's appetite returned, his pain ceased, and his energy level increased. Mr. Malow attributes his pain relief totally to the macrobiotic diet. (This has now been substantiated in other cases that have been relieved of severe spinal pain just several weeks following initiation of the macrobiotic regimen.)

With confirmed return to well-being and improved activity, the patient elected to proceed with diagnostic bone scans. Radiologists at Weiss Memorial Hospital in Chicago found the patient's scans to be markedly improved, and an expert at St. Francis Hospital in Evanston, Illinois, found the recent scans to be "grossly normal." (*Note*: Upon discussion with numerous oncologists in the Evanston/Chicago area, the general opinion was that hormonal therapy would not be a likely explanation for the reversal in Mr. Malow's bone scan.)

The care and improvement seen with this patient, as well as others presently on the same regimen and suffering from metastatic prostate cancer, makes it imperative that serious investigations of this approach be viewed by the medical community without delay.

As President Edward Scanlon of the ACS begins a six-year study to determine life-style effects on cancer development, I urge the general public not to wait for the obvious results. There is a pressing need to promptly change not only our dietary habits, but our life-styles as well. By introducing the macrobiotic approach to health care, we can look forward to a new profile of well-being for the American people.

Below, Mr. Malow exemplifies the feelings of several thousand people who have begun the battle against terminal thinking patterns:

"When I was told I had cancer six years ago, I literally brainwashed myself, refusing to accept the fact that the cancer would overwhelm me. I simply referred to it as my 'little cancer' since I wanted to make it a lesser important evil, rather than a strong all-encompassing, incurable problem. I was told by friends and doctors alike that my positive mental attitude would probably have a great effect regarding the problem of cancer.

"When some friends came across the article by Dr. Sattilaro in the *Saturday Evening Post* regarding his overcoming the very same problems that I have incurred,[1] I proceeded without delay to study and follow the macrobiotic way of life. I am totally convinced that we are what we eat and that we literally destroy our bodies with the poor quality of foods, confections, etc., which we consume. When we analyze the intricate and amazing functions of our body and organs, I further decided we truly should consider the body to be a shrine, which must be given proper nourishment and care.

"At age sixty, despite radiation treatment, some chemotherapy, and other minor problems associated with cancer, I continue to work full time, and also often spend some evening hours doing work. I endeavor to maintain a reasonable amount of exercise and continue to look upon cancer as something that we can overcome with diet and determination. Our amazing bodies apparently can heal themselves if we furnish the body with the proper nourishment, and eliminate that which is harmful."

Thyroid Cancer, Fibroid Tumors

Diane Silver
Thornhill, Ontario, Canada

As a child, I was fed a "balanced diet" (according to modern understanding) and given many vitamin supplements as I grew up. I was sick fairly often as a child; I recall colds, earaches, that kind of thing. I had a very bad case of pneumonia when I was two years old and was given a sulfa drug, which was then in its primi-

---

[1] "An M.D. Who Conquered His Cancer," by Tom Monte, *Saturday Evening Post*, September 1980.

tive stages. I had tonsils and adenoids removed at the age of four. The adenoids grew back, and when I was ten they were removed again by experimental radium treatment.

I had to push myself very hard to keep up with the other students at school in athletics, but I did, and became a very good swimmer. I also led a very active social life. I was teaching school full-time by the time I was nineteen, and was married at twenty. In 1960, a routine examination turned up a very large growing mole on my forehead. It was removed and diagnosed as malignant melanoma.

In 1969 a large fibroid tumor was removed from my uterus. Before that operation, my blood count was down to 30; I hemorrhaged in the hospital, passed out, was declared dead, yet survived! In early 1971 a tumor was found in a lymph node on my neck. I was concerned about melanoma and was relieved when the diagnosis was papillary and follicular carcinoma of the thyroid. My doctor then made two quick moves. He looked up the slides of the pathology report of my malignant melanoma and showed them to a pathologist friend, who declared that to be a somewhat questionable diagnosis. He also sent me off for the removal of my thyroid glands and many other lymph nodes in my neck.

In the years between 1957 and 1971, several other conditions had troubled me. Every few months I would have severe painful cystitis and would be treated with some form of sulfa. I had frequent recurring bouts with pneumonia, for which I received antibiotics regularly. I had a painful troublesome diaphragmatic hernia. I was advised to sleep in a sitting position. I had premenstrual tension, edema, and severe menstrual cramps. I took diuretics and birth control pills.

Between 1971 and 1975, a few more bumps were biopsied from my back and breast, but they were all benign. I was feeling tired and draggy most of the time. I put on 45 extra pounds. My bladder condition and diaphragmatic hernia were troubling me, and I kept getting colds and pneumonia. I had irregular Pap smear tests for three years. I was checked, x-rayed, and scanned for cancer at regular intervals.

By the fall of 1975, I was really sick! My endocrinologist, who also had a fellowship in internal medicine, was very concerned. He decided on a complete series of tests and x-rays for me. After a cystoscopic examination, a urologist declared that I would have to take sulfa for the rest of my life, because there was a stricture in my urethra that was causing chronic infection.

I had an intravenous pyelogram which turned up a shadow on one of my kidneys. Upper and lower gastrointestinal series and scans for cancer showed nothing conclusive. My cholesterol was high, too. But these tests offered no real answers to the constant fatigue and frequent pneumonia bouts. My endocrinologist thought that I had better stop taking the birth control pill. My gynecologist suggested a change of pill, but advised that I should continue that medication because I had growing fibroid tumors that would grow out of control if I stopped.

In late October 1975, I was sick in bed with pneumonia and again on antibiotics. I felt a new lymph node growing on the back of my neck. I rested for weeks with no improvement at all. This sickness seemed very different; I was not getting any better, and my physicians were really stumped.

One day I received a phone call from a pleasant young man named Alan Ginsberg, phoning to deliver regards from a friend of ours in New York. When he heard my gasping and coughing, he remarked, "You sound sick." "Yes, I have pneumonia," I rasped. "What are you eating?" Well, in all my thirty-eight years of life, no physician had ever asked what I was eating.

I told Alan I was eating some cottage cheese, salad, lots of grapefruit and orange juice "because I need fluids." He asked me if I had considered that there were nine to twelve grapefruits in the two or three glasses of juice I was having every day; that grapefruits grow in hot climates—"That this is November and you are in Toronto in the winter and it is getting cold, and furthermore, cottage cheese and all dairy foods create mucus in the body, and you don't need any more mucus!" Was he some kind of nut, I wondered? Or was he making sense?

Was it possible that what I ate could really make a difference in how I felt? I was really very anxious to get well, so I decided to listen. He asked me if I had any whole grains in the house; I only had oatmeal. He advised me to eat just oatmeal, with no milk or sugar on it, for several days, and he would call back. I was terribly skeptical; but after a few days of just oatmeal I was out of bed, feeling better, and ready to listen to what Alan had to say.

He instructed me in the basics of macrobiotics, and I began to read. He also offered treatments to get my energy moving. After a few months I was strong enough to begin a very simple exercise and to take short walks again. I was still skeptical, but I was determined to give it a wholehearted try.

I stopped all medication except the birth control pill and the synthoid. The bladder infection never returned. At the end of December, 1975, Mr. Kushi came to lecture in Toronto and reaffirmed for me everything Alan had said. He amazed me because he diagnosed all my conditions simply by looking at my face and feeling my arm.

Mr. Kushi said that I was still cancerous, and gave me a list of foods to eat and those to avoid. He said I could give up the birth control pill, but not the synthoid. Yet, in February I informed my gynecologist that I was stopping the pill. He assured me that I would be back for a hysterectomy very shortly because the fibroids would grow wildly. The following year at my regular checkup he reported that the fibroids had disappeared, and that I was in better shape than I had been in years. My Pap smear was normal and has remained so. Since then my diaphragmatic hernia has caused no further trouble; my menstrual periods come and go without pain, swelling, or tension at all. I do not get pneumonia any more, although occasionally I cough up phlegm without any sick feeling. There have been no further lumps or bumps. Even the varicose veins in my legs have disappeared.

Last winter, I took up cross country skiing and ice skating again. I used to feel chilled all winter. Now I find pleasure at being outdoors in the cold. My attitude and my body have changed drastically; my entire life has changed for the better.

Uterine and Breast Cancer

Phyllis Crabtree
State College, Pennsylvania

I am a middle aged middle class homemaker, nursery school teacher, wife, mother, and grandmother. In October of 1972, I had an operation for cancer that removed my uterus, Fallopian tubes, and ovaries. In January of 1973 I had a modified radical mastectomy of the right breast. Out of every 100 women who have had those two operations in that sequence, only 15 survive over five years according to statistical prediction.

Why am I still alive? My doctors believe that it is because my operations were performed at such early stages of cancer development. It could be because my son Philip convinced me that it was my responsibility to take care of myself.

He began that campaign many years ago by urging me to eat macrobiotically. He continued by forbidding me to eat any of the hospital foods. He would cook for me at home and bring me *miso* soup, brown rice, and tea in a thermos jug. (The first solid food offered to me by the hospital was Fruit Loops!)

The first time I was admitted, I had to interrupt a teaching schedule. The third time I was an emergency admission on New Year's Day. On Sunday, December 31, 1972, the phone rang at 10 o'clock. The surgeon said that on closer examination the tissue from my right breast and the frozen sections had been negative. I was to be admitted on January 1 and surgery would be done the following day.

When the operations were over, I felt that my body had been mutilated. I did not like my body at all. I felt it had betrayed me by contracting this hideous disease. However, my body and I were still together. I was alive. There was healing to be done.

There was the possibility of my own death to face and work out. I was not ready to die. I wanted to live. Medicine had done all it could for me.

The summer of 1976, my son visited me after an absence of several years and said he had something he wanted to tell me. He chose the airport terminal at the time of his departure.

Briefly, his message was: I was the one who had taken the pills, I was the one who had put the food and the booze and the other medications in my mouth. It was time I took on the responsibility for my own health. What a brash brat, suggesting I was the one who was responsible for my own cancer! I rejected that. I thought it was the doctor's fault, perhaps many doctors' faults.

When I had worked through this idea over and over and over again, my depression finally lessened. Deciding that I could have control over the rest of my life, lessened the feeling of being trapped, the feeling of just waiting helplessly for the cancer to strike again.

Current research says the next place for cancer in women who have been on the pill and estrogen is the liver. I was not looking to join the crowd. In March of 1977, I attended the East West Foundation's Pine Manor conference on cancer in Boston. I listened, and made an appointment with Mr. Kushi. One phrase from the conference kept haunting me: "There are no cancer victims, only cancer producers."

Mr. Kushi recommended a healing diet, and sent me off to eat far more strictly than I had ever eaten before. The fact that his concern was for my liver spurred me to compliance. I attended a summer seminar at Amherst College in 1977 and learned more about myself, food and health; and Mr. Kushi told me that I was getting better. In 1978, I went to the Amherst Program again; Mr. Kushi saw me again and said I was 80 percent healed, but to keep eating carefully. Now, I feel that eating, exercising, and meditation according to the plan suggested by macrobiotics is responsible for my good health.

I am grateful to macrobiotics for more than a cancer cure. For myself there has been an improvement in my aching back caused by osteothorosis, and in chronic urinary infections, both ailments of thirty years' duration. The migraine headaches are fewer in number, less in intensity and duration. Even my motion sickness has lessened.

A diagnosis of cancer is a devastating family event. Care by surgery, x-ray and/or chemotherapy can be traumatic. Convalescence can be difficult. Healing goes on much better in the absence of tension, and in the presence of love.

I had many people helping me, all led by my family. Without them I would not have made it. I thank them and Mr. Kushi.

Cardiovascular Disorders

Cardiovascular Condition, Tension

Jack Saunders
Marblehead, Massachussetts

I was introduced to macrobiotics through a member of a yoga group who had read William Dufty's book, *You Are All Sanpaku.* After reading Dufty's book, I began cooking macrobiotically and attended a few lectures; this was in August of 1971. My colleagues at General Electric definitely considered my diet to be unique, but it never caused me any disruption in my work.

At this time I was very tense, and often found it difficult to deal with people in stressful situations. After eating macrobiotically for only a few weeks, I relaxed quite remarkably, and found I was much more effective in handling difficult situations with people.

The doctors at General Electric had told me I had the beginnings of a cardiovascular condition. Since beginning macrobiotics, this condition has disappeared. Now, I try to work a full day as well as engage in some intense physical activity to activate the entire cardiovascular system. I think this contributes to the health of this vital system, as well as improving my ability to transmute foods. I usually jog, swim, or mountain climb.

I have noticed that while climbing and hiking, my stamina and vitality are very good while eating mostly grains and vegetables, with a small supplement of fish. My colleagues in fact, are often quite impressed by the ability and energy I have with only this simple diet.

I have noticed friends and colleagues my age having various health difficulties, ranging from mild to severe. And without exception, they eat and live in a chaotic fashion, ignoring natural foods and life-style. Even so, I feel that natural foods are not enough; without the guiding principles of yin and yang, natural foods alone cannot insure good health. In fact, I believe the principles of macrobiotics, as applied to both diet and way of thinking, or way of life, are essential in the recovery of good health.

My transition from a standard diet to the macrobiotic diet was gradual and not really very difficult. I simply began to gradually substitute foods as I dropped animal and dairy products. My diet now alters with the season, but basically consists of grains, vegetables, beans, seaweeds, *miso* and *tamari*, and an occasional portion of fish, once a week or so. I have found organic foods are extremely tasty as well as healthful.

I was saying earlier that macrobiotics had a dramatic effect on my ability to work more harmoniously with other people. Shortly after I began the diet, I was instrumental in securing a contract which is still providing a good deal of the work for my General Electric plant in Lynn, Massachusetts. I have found this has become typical, and I really think my diet has aided me in dealing with customers and business. On my previous diet, I was not able to deal as well with people, or to reconcile various differences between people. Macrobiotics has not only changed my physical health; it has changed by entire life.

Heart Disease

Win Donovan
Worthington, Massachussetts
(The following article, written by Tom Monte, is reprinted from the East West Journal.*)*

Win Donovan was trying to remove a large stone from a sewer line when his heart attack struck. Like most people who suffer heart attacks, Donovan's life was radically changed by the devastating blow. Unlike most people whose hearts abruptly stop, though, Donovan says the event changed his life for the better.

On April 27, 1978, Win Donovan was building a house not far from his own home in Worthington in Western Massachusetts. The thirty-eight-year-old contractor owned his construction firm, and at this time, two years before mortgage rates shot up, business was good. In fact, work had been good for the past several years, and Donovan was doing less and less of the tough, physical labor which he had been accustomed to doing before the books were so black. This day was different, however, and Donovan was working hard.

As he struggled with the large rock, he suddenly felt nauseated. A swelling sensation gripped his chest. The swelling changed to pain, which spread from his heart to the rest of his chest and neck. His left arm hurt, and he began to sweat profusely. Donovan had been a volunteer ambulance driver in Worthington and recognized the symptoms. He was scared, but he did not panic.

A friend was standing nearby, and Donovan asked him to ride along to the nearest hospital. They both jumped into Donovan's truck with Donovan behind the wheel. Soon, the pain grew intolerable and he turned over the driving to his friend. Donovan passed out before reaching the emergency room.

Donovan's heart attack did not come as a great surprise. His health had been declining for some time, and by 1975—three years before his heart gave out—he had begun to experience some serious problems. That year, he contracted pneumonia, which left him with pleurisy. He also suffered from extreme kidney trouble. From 1976 until 1978 Donovan had four severe kidney attacks, all of which left him hospitalized and unconscious for days at a time. On top of this, he was discharging red blood cells and protein in his urine. Meanwhile, his cholesterol level hovered at a death-defying 358 mg.; once it reached 395 mg. (Most Americans have cholesterol levels at about 220; anything above 260 is regarded as in the "high risk" range for heart attack or stroke. Heart disease experts regard 180 and below as in the safe range.)

Doctors could not figure out what exactly was wrong with Donovan. According to his physician, Dr. William Shevin, who now practices in Putnam, Connecticut, Donovan had a disease "something on the order of lupus." With all the complications, Shevin says that Donovan was very, very ill. "It's hard to quantify how close anyone is to death," states Shevin, "but Win Donovan was a very sick man."

Donovan was also examined at the Lahey Clinic in Boston, and it was finally decided that he should take antibiotics, cortisone tablets called Prednisone, and diuretics. Nothing worked, however, and Donovan continued to have kidney attacks and recurring pleurisy pain throughout his chest.

While Donovan's health was rapidly declining, his younger brother, Greg, kept telling him about the macrobiotic diet, a regimen consisting mostly of whole grains (brown rice, millet, barley, oats, and corn), beans, vegetables, and seaweed. "I didn't really listen to him," says Donovan today. "You know how it is with younger brothers."

After a while, however, Donovan started listening and made major changes in his diet. However, his practice was haphazard, and he admits today that he had no real understanding of what he was putting in his mouth.

He had been trying to improve his diet for several months when his heart attack came in early April of 1978. When Donovan regained consciousness in the hospital after the attack, his doctors had some bad news. The physicians told him that he would have to make immediate arrangements for a kidney dialysis machine, which he would have to "plug himself" into a couple of times per week in order to go on living. "A kidney machine is temporary," explains Donovan. "You stay with it until you can find a kidney donor for doctors to do a transplant."

Then came the most frightening assessment of his health. "The doctors told me not to make any long-range plans, like taking on any additional debts, because I was not going to be living much longer to pay them off," Donovan recalls.

Shortly thereafter, Donovan made his decision. "It was either decide to take macrobiotics seriously, or take out more life insurance and drive my car off a cliff."

Later that summer, Donovan had another examination with Dr. Shevin. Donovan told Shevin that he had decided to either take another examination with the Lahey Clinic or meet with Michio Kushi, president of the East West Foundation, who was teaching at the Foundation's annual summer program at Amherst College in Amherst, Massachusetts. Shevin, who was familiar with macrobiotics, did not discourage Donovan from going to the Lahey Clinic, but he did encourage him to see Kushi.

"At that point Donovan had decided to take better care of himself," recalls Shevin. "He decided to eat better quality food, cut out smoking and drinking, and seek a higher quality of life. So I encouraged him to do that."

That August, Donovan and his wife went to Amherst but discovered that Kushi's appointments were booked solid. Instead they saw Michael Rossoff, who had been teaching macrobiotics for nearly ten years and had an acupuncture practice with a medical doctor in Rockville, Maryland. When Rossoff saw Donovan, he did not pull any punches.

Rossoff recommended the Standard Macrobiotic Diet—which Donovan says he finally understood for the first time—and some specific recommendations for Donovan's condition.

"He was frightened enough to make dramatic changes in his life," recalls Rossoff, "and his wife was very supportive. That helped him change."

Donovan did not have to wait long to see changes in his condition. "After about a week, I stopped taking all medication," he says. "I was drinking *daikon* radish tea, and that worked as well if not better than the diuretic pills I was taking. The other pills I just stopped."

The pain in his chest, which he had been experiencing regularly, vanished. He stopped having kidney attacks and has not had one since.

Three years of kidney and pleurisy attacks, a heart attack, and weeks in the hospital left Donovan weakened and lethargic. However, within weeks after starting the macrobiotic diet, his strength quickly returned; he began looking again for work.

Donovan returned to see Dr. Shevin shortly thereafter for an examination. "There was a remarkable change in him," says Shevin. "He was still discharging some protein through the urine, but that was a far secondary problem in comparison to the other major improvements he had made."

Shevin recalls that all other signs in Donovan's examination were normal, including pulse rate and blood pressure, both of which were dangerously high before Donovan changed his eating habits.

In September, 1980, Donovan had his blood cholesterol level checked. According to the Beacon Medical Laboratories in Boston, Donovan's cholesterol level today is 200 mg., a drop of nearly 200 mg. from what it was two years ago before he started the macrobiotic diet. Such a steep drop in blood cholesterol indicates that Donovan has sharply reduced one of the major risk factors in heart disease and stroke. Moreover, during those two years, he has taken no medication or therapy, other than maintaining the macrobiotic diet.

Before he started macrobiotics, Donovan weighed 210 pounds. Today he weighs 150. Recently, he tried to cash a money order and used his driver's license as identification. The license bore a photograph of Donovan taken three years ago. The storekeeper looked at him and refused to cash the money order.

Today, Donovan, his wife and two children (a daughter, eighteen, and a son, fourteen) are all practicing macrobiotics. Donovan is once again building houses —with a few variations.

"I used to build about six ranch houses a year. You just throw them together and they go up pretty quick," he says. "Now, I'm building timber frame houses, the kind they used to build 300 years ago. They're better houses and there's a lot more challenge in it."

Donovan wants to build a house that will facilitate and help improve people's health. He also has ideas for developing an air-envelope, solar power kit, which people could assemble themselves or with the aid of a small contractor.

These are major changes for Donovan. However, when asked what the fundamental difference is between the Win Donovan of the past and Win Donovan now, he points to his heart and smiles, "I'm happier today."

Irregular Heartbeat, Fatigue, Insomnia

Lori O'Neil
Ann Arbor, Michigan

My medical history includes constant fatigue since childhood, chronic throat and ear infections, mononucleosis (twice), and anemia. My general condition was never very good.

In November, 1976, I began to develop extreme weakness and dizziness. I began to feel my heart pounding in my chest. The heartbeat was irregular with no pattern, often extremely rapid and pounding hard.

For four months I was unable to work, almost completely bedridden. I was given several medications, tranquilizers, and pain pills for palpitations, insomnia and headaches.

Norpace kept the heartbeat close to normal, but the high dosage I was taking began to cause side effects: constipation, anxiety and insomnia. And I was still very weak and dizzy.

In April, 1977, I returned to work for three hours daily, doing mostly desk work because of my fatigue. By September of that year my condition had not improved at all. While sitting in the waiting room at the University of Michigan Hospital one day, I spoke with an older woman who told me how switching to a vegetarian diet and taking food supplements (vitamins) had cured her of many ailments, including a partially paralyzed arm.

I knew that my diet was not very good, so I was willing to try natural foods to improve my condition. I began by cutting all preservatives, chemicals, meat and sugar out of my diet. I switched to whole grain breads instead of white. I began to eat large amounts of fruits, vegetables, yogurt and nuts, to use honey instead of sugar, and to take multi-vitamin tablets.

Five months later, in February, 1978, I still had shown no improvement. Many times I tried to decrease the amount of medication I was taking for irregular heartbeat, but I could not do it. With any decrease in medication, the discomfort of the irregular heartbeat became unbearable.

In February, I started following the macrobiotic diet and way of life. The diet includes daily whole grains and brown rice, locally grown vegetables as secondary foods, beans, sea vegetables, *miso* or *tamari* soup and occasional cooked fruits as desserts.

Basically, the principle of macrobiotics is to eat organic, locally grown foods as was traditional in most cultures for more than 5,000 years, while making minor adjustments to compensate for seasonal change and present condition. Somewhere in our civilization's past this simple approach to physical and mental health and happiness was lost—I was now recovering it again!

I stopped using dairy products, honey, nuts (except on rare occasion) and vitamins. The macrobiotic diet brought these results: within two or three weeks, my insomnia ended; I began to feel very refreshed in the morning upon awaking. I began to get up earlier, and also to go to sleep earlier at night.

Soon my mental attitude improved and I began to feel generally happier. After about *one month*, my heart began to have less irregular beats; I reduced my dosage of Norpace by one half.

My heart continued to grow stronger, and after *two months* of macrobiotics I stopped taking all medication. At this time my heart was still "skipping" occasionally, but this would not make me feel as light-headed, dizzy or fatigued as before. Also, the pounding feeling in my chest with skipped beats was greatly reduced.

During the next six weeks (after stopping medication) I began to feel stronger very quickly. I felt much more energetic, and palpitations were few. I began to exercise much more, as it was springtime and I was spending much time outdoors. I was no longer held back by any symptoms. With a group of friends, I was able to keep up in any sport or activity.

I can describe my present condition as one of continuous improvement. Any palpitations I have experienced have been minor and infrequent. I have also overcome other difficulties and experienced additional benefits since starting macrobiotics. Among them is a great change in personality: I used to be a quiet type of person, uncomfortable with strangers, even withdrawn, and always tried to avoid social get-togethers, strangers and meeting new people. Now I love being with people, am more confident and comfortable with all people and welcome making new friends.

I have learned that you cannot separate the mind and the body. They are one. And both are affected by what you eat and drink daily.

I am now responsible for my own health, and I feel this is the way it was intended to be. I will continue to study macrobiotics and to adjust my diet according to my condition, to keep myself in the greatest possible state of health, both physically and mentally.

Miscellaneous

Miscellaneous Disorders

Keith Block, M.D.

Below I have briefly summarized a small group of patients that I have worked with in terms of specific illnesses and their improvements through change to the macrobiotic approach. I am only placing emphasis on the specific ailments the patient came in for, although many other problems have cleared up with each of these patients.

Patient No. 1 Anthony Deppong—Terminal Brain Tumor (Dysgerminoma)
This eighteen-year-old gentleman was diagnosed in April 1979 with a pituitary beta cell adenoma. He underwent surgery and radiation treatments, in which his parents were informed that the tumor was a dysgerminoma and was found to be inoperable. He underwent further surgery for ventricular shunts, a craniotomy, and was placed on several medications including chemotherapy and steroids.

Mr. and Mrs. Deppong visited me in August of 1981 and acknowledged their drive from Wisconsin was a last hope. At this time Anthony's tumor had obstructed the shunts placed in his head during the last surgery due to the tumor's large size. According to Mrs. Deppong, chemotherapy had not been helping so the Wisconsin doctors elected to begin radiation. They clearly did not feel that this would help due to the massive tumor size, and two of the doctors gave them no hope at all. Along with the radiation therapy the pediatrician-oncologist and pediatrician welcomed any help that the diet would give. They only asked that the diet be reviewed by the hospital dietician (St. Mary's Hospital, Madison, Wisc.). The dietician's comment after reviewing the diet was, "Go to it, it is a good diet and Anthony will get everything he needs from it."

After beginning the macrobiotic diet Anthony experienced progressive improvement in his energy, vitality, memory, and appetite. In December 1981 Mrs. Deppong called me to report, "After a CAT scan was done, the surgeon said there was no sign of the tumor anywhere in his head . . . and the pediatrician said that they had hoped to see a reduction in the tumor size but to find it absolutely gone had to be a miracle."

Anthony, his parents, and my personal feeling is that the diet was the responsible factor in causing the tumor to disappear. Mrs. Deppong says, "I strongly urge everyone to get on the macrobiotic diet. It may be difficult at first, and it is a whole different life-style, but it is well worth it. All of us feel so good, and now we really do not even want to go off it. Also we have made such friends that are true, true friends among the macrobiotic community."

According to Anthony, "I am energetic and I am now playing tennis twice a week. Recently I saw a television commercial on sugar cereals. It made me sad for people who just do not know. I got up and ran to my mother and gave her a big hug. I thanked her for putting us on the macrobiotic diet. These days I am so happy and experiencing so much energy. It feels great!"

Patient No. 2   Allan Schulman—Arthritis, Colitis

This forty-seven-year-old gentleman presented with osteoarthritis in the neck with marked cervical spurs. He also suffered significant pain in the sacral region (lower back), along with regular bouts of active colitis for the past twenty years. One month after beginning the macrobiotic diet and regular massage therapy his arthritic pain improved. He also acknowledged improvement with his colitis. Within three months after initiation of the macrobiotic way of life, Mr. Schulman acknowledged "feeling terrific" with regard to his once diagnosed arthritis and colitis. In his words: "I suffered for maybe twenty years with colitis and the last two years I had begun to develop arthritis in my neck and hands. Within a week of going on the diet, I stopped taking my daily doses of liquid antacid. For eight months I have been adhering to the diet as closely as I can combining it with exercises for my neck and back. My colitis seems to have disappeared and the arthritis is responding dramatically. When I do not follow the diet as closely as I should I can almost immediately notice the difference in how I feel."

Patient No. 3   Mary Theresa Gleason—Asthma, Allergies, Colitis

This thirty-four-year-old woman presented with complaints of several years of chronic bronchial asthma. Over the week prior to her visit, she suffered from two severe attacks of coughing, wheezing, and breathing difficulties (shortness of breath). After having tried numerous preparations in the past, including homeopathic remedies, we began her on a macrobiotic regimen, and withdrew all previous preparations. Over the following months, she showed progressive improvement. Occasionally during that time, she experienced recurrences only when she went off the specific macrobiotic program recommended for her. The foods that aggravated her condition were milk and dairy products, flour products, nut butters, and sweets. Over the following several months of refining her macrobiotic practice, she has markedly improved. At this time she has not experienced any attacks for the duration of sixteen months. In her words: "Over the past twenty years I experienced bronchial asthma, allergies and severe attacks of colitis. The bronchial asthma was progressively worsening. I saw several dozen medical doctors, was hospitalized and visited emergency rooms numerous times during these years. Also I was placed on different asthmatic inhalants, brochosol, epinephrine, various diets, and was told to keep oxygen at home. Since Dr. Block put me on the macrobiotic diet in June of 1981 I have had no problems with my asthma, allergies or colitis. The only time that I have had even a little wheezing is when I have gone off his specific recommendations. In fact, when I eat macrobiotically and stay away from flour products and sweets, I really have no problems at all."

Patient No. 4   Lindell Thorsen—Renal Vascular Hypertension
This twenty-eight-year-old woman presented with renal vascular hypertension that was diagnosed medically in 1977. On presentation to my office, she was taking Inderal and Dyazide in order to control her blood pressure. Her pressure at the time of initial appointment was 150 systolic over 113 diastolic with medications. One month after beginning the standard macrobiotic program, her pressure came down to within normal limits. All medications were stopped and her pressure remained at that level. Over one year later the patient still maintains a normal blood pressure without medications and continues the macrobiotic diet.

Patient No. 5   Camilee Baranchick—Duodenal Ulcer/Sinusitis (Severe)
This thirty-six-year-old woman presented on December 11, 1981, suffering from severe painful duodenal ulcers without active bleeding or melena (black stool). This condition started in 1968; after which she saw several physicians over the next decade with repeated suggestion of various medications and surgery.

The patient was also suffering from continuous sinusitis and post-nasal drip. During the first month of macrobiotic practice, her ulcer pain improved dramatically and her sinus condition cleared up as well. However, during the first six weeks of practice she would occasionally widen her diet with the return of symptoms. Upon resuming the standard diet, her condition would again clear up. With steady improvement over the next several months, Mrs. Baranchick has cured her condition.

According to her: "After fourteen years of unsuccessful treatment with the conventional medical ulcer diet, I have finally found a way to relieve my pain. In August, Dr. Block prescribed a macrobiotic dietary plan and within two weeks I began to feel dramatic relief. Besides this, for the three years prior to my visit I suffered from severe sinusitis. At that time I underwent two operations that were both debilitating and unsuccessful. The problem continued until I changed my diet and then the condition cleared up almost instantaneously. Six months after following Dr. Block's initial recommendations, I have continued to experience a life without these debilitating problems. My energy and total well-being have improved daily and the entire experience has been marvelous. I attribute this to the macrobiotic program."

Patient No. 6   Linda Haberkorn—Myasthenia Gravis
This thirty-year-old woman was diagnosed at eighteen years old with myasthenia gravis. At the time of her initial office visit the patient was taking 90 mg. of Mestinon every four hours. Within the next few months, Mrs. Haberkorn has shown marked improvement in her condition with a reduction in medication. In her words: "Since starting on a macrobiotic diet I have been able to reduce my medication by one half and I have much more energy and vitality than before. Prior to the diet I tried to reduce my medicine but was always forced to return to the original dosage. When I am following Dr. Block's recommendations more closely my condition seems to disappear. I am confident that due to macrobiotics I will eventually be able to stop my medications completely. I recommend this diet for all myasthenia gravis patients. It has helped me enormously."

Patient No. 7   Shannon Battaglia—Severe Otitis Media (Severe Ear Infection with Drainage), Swollen Lymph Nodes

Four-and-a-half-year-old child presented with three months of purulent left ear drainage (whitish pus). This continuous drainage had been treated unsuccessfully with numerous preparations prior to initial appointment. At the time of presentation, the patient also suffered from active tonsillitis. Within one week of the standard macrobiotic regimen, there was complete clearing of the ear drainage with significant improvement in the tonsil condition. According to her mother:

"Our family was vegetarian when Shannon became ill. We ate a diet high in dairy, cheese, butter, yogurt, tropical fruits and fruit juices, tomato sauces, and a lot of flour products (breads, etc.). At age two she developed asthma and was told to stop dairy. This helped but only temporarily. She frequently had coughs, colds, and wheezing.

"In the winter of 1980–81, Shannon developed a severe draining ear infection with very swollen glands. We tried numerous preparations and finally decided to see Dr. Block. On our visit he diagnosed Shannon by using visual diagnosis and then confirmed this through looking in her ears and throat. He told us to follow a specific version of the macrobiotic diet for her particular problems which included two teaspoons of *azuki* beans daily and the strict avoidance of flour products, fruits, sweets, and excess oil for two weeks. Within four days her swollen glands and ear infection began clearing up. Now whenever Shannon gets any signs of a cold or runny nose we get strict again and she gets better immediately."

Patient No. 8   Sara Crawford—Infantile Baldness

This adorable two-year-old girl presented to my office in April of 1981 suffering from idiopathic infantile alopecia (infantile baldness with unknown cause) and chronic urinary tract infections. She saw numerous medical specialists and tried several medications, all to no avail. Within one week after beginning the Standard Macrobiotic Diet, with an emphasis on sea vegetables (due to her severe mineral depletion), new hair growth began over her balding head. Her urinary tract infections subsided as well. Today she is a happy, healthy macrobiotic child with a beautiful head of hair.

Patient No. 9   Herbert Nussbaum—Osteoarthritis, Bursitis

This fifty-seven-year-old gentleman presented with several years of osteoarthritis and bursitis to the shoulders and neck region. Shortly after beginning the standard macrobiotic regimen Mr. Nussbaum experienced significant relief of pain and dramatic improvement in range of motion in his upper extremities. Over the next few months, his condition markedly improved.

Patient No. 10   Deborah Senn—Recurrent Bladder and Vaginal Infections

This thirty-three-year-old woman has suffered for several years of chronic recurring bladder and vaginal infections. After trying numerous medications and developing a secondary yeast infection she presented to my office. She was placed on a Standard Macrobiotic Diet with specific recommendations and adjustments to treat her particular condition. Shortly thereafter these infections cleared up. In her words: "As long as I stick to the dietary recommendations Dr. Block has made I have no difficulties. In fact my entire well-being is improved while sticking to the macrobiotic diet."

Patient No. 11   Mary Willis—Fertility Problem
This thirty-one-year-old woman presented to my office in March, 1981, having tried unsuccessfully to become pregnant for over one year. Having felt that there was some problem with ovulation we began a macrobiotic regimen. By June of 1981 Mrs. Willis, feeling "terrific" since her initiation on the program, became pregnant. On March 17, she delivered a beautiful baby boy.

According to Mrs. Willis: "When I first saw Dr. Block concerning my fertility problem I had no idea of the dietary benefits I would experience. My energy level tripled and I could go an entire day without becoming tired. My mental attitude became hopeful and positive as well. Several months after beginning the macrobiotic diet I became pregnant. The diet was very difficult at first but as the weeks went by it became much easier. Now I enjoy the diet very much and my earlier resistance has dissipated. Also, my general well-being has improved and I feel fortunate to be on the macrobiotic diet and am grateful for Dr. Block's assistance."

Patient No. 12   Betty Lubach—Glaucoma
Forty-nine-year-old white female diagnosed with glaucoma in 1976. Began macrobiotic diet November 1979 with intraocular pressures of 31 in both eyes. Within three months, Mrs. Lubach's pressures dropped to 23 then 21, far below the dangerous condition she originally had. Mrs. Lubach's eye specialist later desired to change her diagnosis to intraocular hypertension, a milder form of the original disease. After careful scrutiny with him, the patient was able to get him to leave his original diagnosis of glaucoma. Since modern medicine says there is no cure, he felt his diagnosis was incorrect. However, it is rather obvious that her condition has drastically improved due to these dietary changes. This should be considered a cure for this once felt incurable disorder.

Patient No. 13   Jimmy Ilson—Juvenile Onset Diabetes
Twenty-one-year-old white male. Mr. Ilson was diagnosed with and has been suffering from juvenile onset diabetes mellitus for over a decade. After seeing Mr. Ilson, his parents still insisted that he enter Joslin Clinic in Boston, Mass. to be regulated on his insulin level. Mr. Ilson was able to stay in the hospital for the eight-day visit with full cooking facilities and stayed on the diet throughout this period. His level changed dramatically during his first week on the diet. His original insulin requirement declined by two-thirds during that time. Both doctors and nutritionists remarked how unusual such an occurrence is. In fact, a leading nutritionist at Joslin claimed that the macrobiotic diet was obviously the future diet for diabetics everywhere.

Patient No. 14   Robin Cole—Pelvic Inflammatory Disease
Twenty-six-year-old white female. Mrs. Cole presented to my office after her second bout with pelvic inflammatory disease. The patient initially was diagnosed with a large baseball size right tubo-ovarian abscess and surgery was suggested. The patient was treated with intravenous fluids but avoided surgery and went home from the hospital only to return one month later. After her second hospitalization with repeat surgical recommendations and refusal, the patient was referred to me. I placed her on a Standard Macrobiotic Diet with regular applications of hot ginger compresses to the abscessed right ovary. Within three weeks after beginning this therapy, the patient returned to her original gynecologist who announced to the patient and her own surprise that the abscess was gone. Since that time the patient has remained on the Standard Macrobiotic Diet without any further difficulties.

Patient No. 15   Dolores Harmon—Kidney Stone
Forty-nine-year-old white female. Mrs. Harmon was referred to me following refusal to undergo surgery on a left kidney stone that had not passed after intravenous fluid and medications while hospitalized in June 1980. X-rays demonstrating the stone are available from June 9, 10, and 13. A Standard Macrobiotic Diet with twice daily applications of hot ginger compresses to the left kidney were done for three full weeks. The patient's pain subsided dramatically during the third week of treatment and on July 3, 1980, an x-ray series was taken which was consistent with passage of the once lodged renal stone.

Miscellaneous Disorders

Compiled by the East West Foundation, Brookline, Massachussetts and the Community Health Foundation, London

Allergies—Bill Tims, Tulsa, Oklahoma
Before I was seven years old I had many earaches and sore throats. As it was the common suggestion of doctors, I decided that removing my tonsils would eliminate the source of these problems, because they were continually becoming inflammed. (I never considered their inflammation a natural bodily defense against poisons entering my system.) Shortly after having this tonsillectomy I began to develop more and more intense allergies. Each time I had a violent sneezing attack, my parents and I decided upon some *obvious* external cause: weeds, sunflowers, cats, dust, etc. However, as time went by, it seemed as though the number of things I was allergic to was growing larger and larger, until I found myself surrounded by an alien world. My natural environment was mysterious and often evil when causing me to sneeze *without any reason at all*.

   As my allergies appeared and left with the changing seasons, I was dealing with a much deeper sickness within myself. Sometimes conscious, sometimes unconscious, never talked about with friends, was a vacancy within myself, a lack of vitality. School did not offer solutions to this. Church did not offer solutions to this. Sometimes I felt alive with friends, only to realize when I was alone that it had been their efforts and not mine. I can remember going hunting with my father and watching his bird-dogs run all day long, up and down gulleys, across meadows and fields, disappearing and reappearing, never tiring. That hunger, that sense of search and adventure, was what I wanted to feel in my heart. Overweight, lazy, lacking challenge and initiative, I passively assumed any role necessary for coping with various social situations.

Amidst all this there came to me a ragged copy of a book entitled the *Book of Judgment* by George Ohsawa, which introduced a way of life called macrobiotics. It made complete, stunning sense to me. In a very short time, through good friends I found out that a man named Michio Kushi had studied with Mr. Ohsawa and was teaching macrobiotics in Boston. I came to Boston to study with him. Among other things, he told me that my over-consumption of dairy foods, sugar and liquids were the major causes of my allergies and excess weight. He suggested that I eliminate these from my diet and begin to take grains, vegetables, beans and seaweeds as my principal foods. After two months of following his recommendations, I had lost 30 pounds and in six months my allergies were under complete control. Over the years I have begun to feel an intense aliveness within myself, surging and radiating at the roots. I find that I can share and develop understanding with friends, without our relationships being consumed in too many thoughts or emotions. To these friends, to my parents who have always tried to teach me native common sense I am grateful. I am also grateful to Mr. Ohsawa and Mr. Kushi for a glimpse at the infinite universe and its unifying principle of yin and yang, whereby I can carry on my life and my study with order and direction.

Arthritis—Marty Kalan, Philadelphia, Pennsylvania

I was diagnosed as arthritic in both hands (in about seven fingers) by a doctor in Philadelphia. At the time of diagnosis, he said, "Look, let's verify it. Go get x-rays and let's see what we find." I had x-rays taken and of course verified that I was arthritic. It was very painful. I asked the doctor what could be done about it. He said, "I'm sure you know there's no cure for arthritis." I told him I thought it was awful that the medical profession had no cure for arthritis, and asked what I could do. He suggested that I take pain relievers—aspirin, etc. I asked if that was all there was to it. He said, "Yes, that's what everybody else does." I left and forgot about it. That was about ten years ago.

About eight years ago, I was in Israel with my son, walking up a hill huffing and puffing. He asked what was wrong and I answered that I was getting old, fifty-four-years old, and was slowing down. He said, "Nonesense, why don't you stop eating that bad food that you've been eating." I said, "What do you mean?" He answered, "You know, get into macrobiotics, like me." I said, "I don't want to eat your stuff. You mean no steak, no meat?" He said, "Just stop eating refined sugars, cake, candy, and ice cream, like you have been eating, and cut out some of the meat." He asked how many times a week I ate meat and I realized that

I must have eaten it twice a day. Every dinner, and for lunch, and a midnight snack. I must have eaten meat from eighteen to twenty times a week. He told me to reduce my meat intake and to stop eating sugar.

After two weeks, I began feeling a little better. I was a greeting card salesman at that time and I used to get dizzy spells after walking two or three blocks. My bags weighed about 40 pounds, and I could not understand it. But after these two or three weeks that started to disappear. And as the months went on my bowels started getting better. I used to be fearful of going into the bathroom. I used to go in and read a paper and just had such a terrible time. But now by comparison—I will bring my story up to date because I could go on for hours— my fingers are without pain. I have no apparent arthritis at all. I can squeeze and massage my fingers with no pain at all.

My eyes have also improved. I used to wear my glasses about 90 percent of the time, and 10 percent would not wear them. I would not wear them for distance. I am wearing my glasses today about 10 percent of the time, and do not wear them about 90 percent. Plus, I have no more dizzy spells. On the contrary, I can run a mile or two now.

My pulse rate has gone from about 76 to 64. I can play 2, 3, 4, 5 sets of singles in tennis and think nothing of it; play with my son who is thirty-year-old and my son-in-law who is thirty-two and hold my own. Macrobiotics has changed my life completely. I am happier, I hear better, and although I am not trying to lose weight, I have lost about 35 pounds in the last seven-and-a-half years of macrobiotics. I have been eating about 60 percent grains, 30 percent vegetables, beans, *miso* soup every day, etc. Occasionally I binge and if I do, it discharges. It might come out as a little pimple or something.

I had a very bad back and that improved tremendously. I feel that macrobiotics is the best thing that has ever happened to me in my life. I am sixty-one-year-old, going on sixty-two. I am so pleased and so humbly grateful for this program that my son put me onto. Of course, I call it the Michio Kushi macrobiotic program, and it certainly is a change of life for me. My way of life has changed, and God only knows so much for the better, and I really and truly feel terrific.

Arthritis, Varicose Veins—Patricia Goodwin, Revere, Massachusetts

I have been macrobiotic for seven years. I discovered this way of life while working as a waitress in a macrobiotic restaurant in Boston. I was not seriously ill before beginning macrobiotics, but I had many ailments. I can list them as physical: arthritis and varicose veins, and psychological: anger, depression, and extreme self-consciousness.

Since high school I had been feeling pain from arthritis, later diagnosed as "tendency toward rheumatoid arthritis" by Dr. Crowley of Lynn, Massachusetts in approximately 1971. The stiffness was present in almost every joint in my body, but most especially in my hands, shoulders and back. Such daily tasks as carrying books, reaching or bending were uncomfortable. At times no movement was necessary to bring a dull, persistent ache to my back. The doctor took x-rays and prescribed darvon and aspirin three times a day. Every time I went to the office the nurse would question me. Did I have headaches? Did the pain keep me awake at night? These questions worried me, because I thought they expected me to get worse. The medication did not help. After a couple of weeks I discontinued it and the office visits as well. I went on as before, ignoring my condition or enduring it, depending on the strength of the pain.

Another problem I had had was varicose veins, which, like the arthritis, were considered by me and my family to be inherited and therefore impossible to cure. The pain consisted of a tenderness and throbbing in the swollen veins, sometimes sharp enough to make walking difficult. Operations and drugs were foreseen in the future.

After just a few months of eating macrobiotically my arthritic condition began to improve. I forgot about the constant pain and stiffness of arthritis until one day when I ate some cheese and drank some wine. Right away I felt the old, familiar pain in my back. I then realized that the pain I had lived with for so long, not only had disappeared, but most certainly had been caused by my imbalanced eating. I do not take such extreme foods now, and the pain of arthritis has disappeared completely.

The varicose veins have pretty much disappeared. Only one, which was always the largest, of the swollen veins remains. I never feel any pain or throbbing from it and I never have any trouble walking.

Diabetes—Ken Becker, Reston, Virginia

About nine years ago, I began to look for alternatives to the conventional medical way of treating my diabetic condition, which I had had for about six years. I found it hard to accept the conclusion that because of my condition, I would have to live my whole life as a *sick* man. A little over six years ago, my search was rewarded: I discovered macrobiotics, a system that not only offered me hope, but actually started to heal me in front of my own eyes!

I undertook macrobiotics as a skeptic, and only my own practical experiences have convinced me of its effectiveness. The thing that impressed me most about macrobiotics was not only that it *worked*, but that it provided me with an explanation of *why* I had diabetes—something conventional medicine had been unable to do—and of how my body would react and change as it began to heal itself. I was amazed at how accurate these predictions were. In eight months, just as predicted, my body's requirement of insulin was reduced by one half, from about 40–42 units per day to about 18–20 units per day.

Even more impressive was the dramatic improvement in my overall health. As any medical doctor and every diabetic knows, diabetes has an effect on the person's general health: circulation is impeded, susceptibility to colds and infections increases, eyesight deteriorates, muscle tone is harder to maintain, and so forth. Before becoming diabetic, I was a fairly healthy child. Afterward, I watched as my health deteriorated in these and many other ways. All of these complications have disappeared since I have become macrobiotic, and my general good health is returning.

I have not had a cold since becoming macrobiotic (my previous average was four to five times per year), a seven times per year case of red, sore throat has disappeared (my doctor had told me "that's just the way you are"), a seven times per year long case of running nose has vanished, my eyesight has improved, I have no more headaches, my gums no longer bleed when I brush my teeth, my previously poor complexion is a thing of the past, I no longer get muscle cramps and nervous twitches—the list could go on and on. Some of these improvements could be attributed to the improvement in my diabetic condition, but I believe they are all directly related to my change in eating.

Diabetes—Peter Howes, Hertfordshire, England

I went to the Community Health Foundation in London in September 1977 to talk about my diabetic condition, and was given a specific macrobiotic diet to follow. The difficulties of preparing the macrobiotic meals were overcome by gradually incorporating the new foods into our normal family diet. After four weeks I was completely on the new diet, and found the transition from the established habits of a lifetime much easier than I had anticipated. At first I experienced some stomach pains, but these have not recurred.

I occasionally craved for the foods I used to enjoy. (I would wake up in the night with my mouth watering at the thought of dried fruits, oranges and bananas!) But these cravings soon passed, and now the only remaining desire is for an occasional glass of beer. I do not give into this, though, for fear of once again becoming a drinker, with the accompanying problem of excess liquid.

The most amazing development over the last nine months has been a new state of quietness and calm. My sleeping habits have also become more regular: I am usually in bed by 11: 00 P.M., and awake completely refreshed at 5: 30 A.M. Before my change in diet I was useless until 10: 00 A.M. (and my first cup of coffee—on which I was dependent throughout the day!).

Now, about nine months after beginning macrobiotics, my insulin requirement has been reduced by about one half, and I find that my condition is easier to control, since the tendency to swing from high blood sugar to low blood sugar has been stabilized by my new diet. My weight has also reduced, and I feel very fit and full of energy.

Endometriosis—Dawn Gilmour, Edinburgh, Scotland

When I was seventeen years of age I went to the doctor with pain in my back and sides. I also had extremely painful menstruation which had gone on for several years. A blood test and urine samples were taken, but nothing could be found, and I was put on antibiotics and pain killers. In 1969, I went into the hospital for one month with nephritis. Then, in 1972, after complaining for a number of years about the same pain and having been in the hospital four times for observation, I was told that my condition was probably psychosomatic. My doctors also told me that they would "open me up to keep me quiet," and when they did, they found that I had acute appendicitis and a cyst on the right ovary.

I never did feel right after that operation. I became very weak and continued going into the hospital for investigations (D and C), and was continually on antibiotics.

In 1976 it was discovered that I had endometriosis. I also had ovarian cysts and blocked Fallopian tubes. My surgeon, one of the leading female gynecologists in Scotland, tried to persuade me to have a hysterectomy. I was only twenty-four, and was told that with all of the trouble I had had, "it was just useless baggage." I really had to battle with the surgeon not to have the hysterectomy. During the operation my tubes were cut and "unblocked," and cysts and tissue from the endometriosis were removed. I was then given heat treatment because it was felt that I was not healing quickly enough. Large electric pads were placed on the ovary region. These pads conducted tremendous heat, and I stopped after four treatments because it was causing blisters on my skin and excessive bleeding.

I then went for a second opinion. The surgeon who I saw was shocked at my condition and could not believe that I was still walking around. I was sent immediately to the hospital for rest and observation. This new doctor said that heat treatment should not be used for my condition as it would accelerate the endometriosis. So in 1977, surgery was performed to remove the left Fallopian tube which had collapsed. Cysts were also removed from the ovaries.

I was then put on hormone treatments so as to suppress all menstruation, as this was believed to be a factor in spreading the endometriosis. One month after this operation I had a pelvic abcess and was rushed by ambulance to the hospital. They could not operate as it was too dangerous. I was placed in intensive care. I was given blood transfusions, could not urinate, and had tubes everywhere. The doctor did not think I would live. After two weeks the abcess burst and began to drain through the bowel. Little did I know that this would mean I would be running to the toilet up to nine times a day for the next month.

I stayed on the hormones for nine months and then decided to stop taking them. I was having severe headaches and pains in my kidneys, and had gone from 91 to 128 1bs. My heart felt very strained. I had no energy and looked like a walking balloon.

In 1978 I went back into the hospital for an investigation to see how things were going. I really felt no difference. It turned out that everything had accelerated and I was back to square one. The surgeon looked at me and said, "I don't know what to say."

During these years of illness I had tried many alternative approaches to healing, including acupuncture, homeopathy, herbs, and faith healing. I had also tried eating a vegetarian diet since 1972. Nothing seemed to make any long term difference. I had also seen psychiatrists and was classed as a manic depressive.

I then met a friend who told me about macrobiotics. I decided to go to London to see Mr. Kushi. I felt I could not do any more damage by trying something else. I was so desperate to get well—to feel human again.

Mr. Kushi gave me certain dietary recommendations which I followed. I felt a difference within four days. Physically, I knew it was going to take a little time to get well, but the change in my mental attitude was so dramatic, so quick, I could hardly believe it. It was an overwhelming transformation for me, and my husband was thrilled with his "new wife."

Nine months later I went back to the Royal Infirmary for another internal examination. No endometriosis was found. My doctor, who had performed my previous surgery, thought that my recovery was unbelievable; he was so happy for me and encouraged me to continue on the macrobiotic diet as that seemed to be the thing that was changing my condition.

My last checkup was in September of 1981, just before I moved to Boston. I had an internal examination and Pap smear. Again, the results showed no problems.

I am so grateful to Mr. Kushi, to my husband who supported me continuously, and to all my friends for their support, Without their compassion and encouragement things would have been so difficult. We must have this support, faith, and determination, and must realize that we are responsible for our own health and that we have the ability to change everything.

Epilepsy (Petit Mal)—Joe Avoli, East Templeton, Massachusetts

Since I can remember, I always had some sort of problems, usually small. However, in the fifth grade, I was out of school for three consecutive weeks with an illness which was very unusual, at least to me. One week, I had measles and another I had scarlet fever and the last week I had poison ivy. I was stiff from the poison ivy and in such pain and irritation, that I felt I could only have been worse off if I had been covered with burns since my skin had a burning irritating itch.

Another thing which plagued me was anemia, at times I would have plenty of energy and at other times I wished someone would carry me home from school. I just did not have the energy to walk home without a lot of effort. I can also remember at times getting heart palpitations, but only when eating sugar donuts or other sugar products, which also caused great depressive states in me. I would feel that life in general was going so poorly, that it was just a real chore at best to live and not really worth it.

I also had petit mal epilepsy, which is a small seizure (fainting spells) along with vertigo which is dizziness upon arising. I was given a brain scan (EEG) electroencephalogram, and put on three tablets of dilantin per day for the rest of my life, as far as the doctors knew. These pills always made me tired, especially early at night. It was difficult for me to stay up late on certain occasions and I would feel guilty about falling asleep or going to bed early. I also bit my nails constantly and sometimes they would bleed and be sore for the longest time. I had an explosive temperament too, which got me into trouble more than once and kept my friends limited.

After years of all of this nonsense (especially the twelve years of taking medication for the aforementioned epilepsy), I said to my wife, "This is crazy, and I'm going to throw this stuff out." I did and I have never taken any medication since. This was ten years ago, at the time of beginning macrobiotics. The first ten days of the diet were educational and therapeutic. At the end of ten days, I had no more anemia, and I could stay awake until twelve o'clock at night, and then go to sleep in five minutes with perfect rest after six hours.

That for me was a big change and I also awoke ready to spring up and become active. After a couple of months of good eating, I had no more dizziness upon arising from a chair or whatever (vertigo) and I stopped biting my nails, gradually, and they became stronger. Before this, my nails would crack and they were soft. I have never had another seizure since, nor even slight dizziness.

I am not subject to depression any more and even find myself calm under pressure, unless I eat something which produces the opposite effect. It has been at least nine years since my last palpitation, and I never get poison ivy now, unless I break the plant and get the juice on me, and even then it is cured quickly by narrowing the diet.

When you have had experiences like this, you can really see how food makes sickness or not. All of these troubles I have had I can undeniably see as caused by food, which is taken for granted and abused by so many people. I am grateful for this life, which has come from food, good food, macrobiotic food without which I probably would soon be ready for some kind of mental institution, according to my past. I also thank George Ohsawa infinitely, and Michio Kushi and others spreading macrobiotics so dedicatedly for so many years. I hope many people try it, I am sure they will find it as indelible as I have.

Epilepsy—Helen Lincoln, Gwynedd, England

I first began to experience the symptoms of epilepsy when I was fourteen. From that time on, I went through the usual procedure: specialists in London hospitals, drugs and psychiatrists. Not one doctor could say why I suddenly started to suffer from epilepsy. I was put on Phenobarbitone, which made me very depressed, and consequently had to take anti-depressant tablets. I was then put on Mysoline, but it did not control my attacks, which became more severe as I entered my twenties.

At the age of twenty-two I was married, and my husband was a great boost to my morale. He took me to see other specialists and psychiatrists, but to no avail. At this time I was on 250 mg. of Mysoline per day, and my husband was constantly receiving telephone calls from hospitals saying that I was under their care after being found in an attack.

My first child was born in April 1965, my second in November 1966. I was not allowed to have any more children, owing to complications, which was just as well as my epilepsy was still severe. I never actually hurt the children, though I did do some damage to myself several times.

Several years after the birth of my children I became a vegetarian. This diet was a little help, but was not by any means a complete answer. My husband said I used to have two or three attacks in the night, and I would occasionally have one during the day. These would begin about the time of menstruation and continue over three or four days.

In the autumn of 1974, I happened to buy a book on macrobiotic cooking. After studying it for a couple of days, I felt it was the diet I had been looking for. I was not thinking of my epilepsy so much as of my general health. I found further books on macrobiotics, and started applying the philosophy they taught.

My attacks became infrequent, and they ceased altogether within twelve months. In 1977, when I had been without an attack for two years, I asked my doctor if

I could stop taking my daily Mysoline doses. He was rather skeptical, but sent me for an EEG test (of which I have had many over the past years.) He was amazed at the result—all signs of epilepsy had disappeared. I gradually cut down the Mysoline at first, then eliminated it altogether.

My change of diet has also affected my whole attitude to life. Both my concentration and my memory have improved considerably. My general health is good, and coupled with the fact that I no longer have epileptic seizures, my self-confidence has returned. I used to find it difficult to wake up after eight, ten or twelve hours of sleep; I now sleep six hours, on the average, and rise about six o'clock every morning.

To sum up—I suffered from severe epilepsy for over twenty-five years, just managing to cope with the necessities of life. I have been macrobiotic for nearly four years, during the first year of which my attacks ceased altogether. I am now able to cope with two children, a part-time job, a large house and garden. My physical and mental health are excellent, and I lead a very full and varied life.

Multiple Sclerosis—Doreen Cassidy, Blackpool, England

About seven years ago I noticed that the first finger and thumb of my right hand became numb. This numbness gradually spread to all of my right hand, resulting in an inability to feel any sensations in that hand. About three months later, I developed double vision in both eyes. I was referred to a specialist at Blackpool General Hospital, where I stayed for about ten days. During this period I was given massive doses of cortisone every day. The double vision began to get better, and after a month the condition vanished.

A few months later I suddenly found that my entire right side was numb; this happened almost overnight. I was then referred to a neurologist at Preston, who said that I had a spinal nervous disorder, but gave me no treatment. I saw him once a year for the next five years. During this period I began to develop a limp in my right leg and a twitching which gradually became worse. I was given a lumbar puncture, but was told that there was "nothing wrong."

One day in April 1977, I got up in the morning and found I had no feeling from the waist down. I got in touch with my doctor and was referred to a specialist who confirmed that I had multiple sclerosis.

I was again given massive doses of cortisone. This time I was only able to walk very slowly, with the aid of two walking sticks. My legs felt as if they were going to burst, and being on my legs was extremely painful.

While I was ill I learned of the Community Health Foundation through my husband's boss at work. I immediately contacted the Foundation and was told that Michio Kushi was then in London. An appointment was arranged for me. On May 10, 1977, I went down to London, where I had to be carried upstairs to see Mr. Kushi; he told me that I could be helped by macrobiotics. I stopped the cortisone and commenced the new way of eating straight away.

Within three or four weeks my walking became much less difficult and my balance gradually improved. The numbness also disappeared. On March 20, 1978, I went for a second visit with Mr. Kushi. This time my improvement had been so considerable that I was able to walk up four flights of stairs using only one walking stick. My diet was varied by cutting out fruit and reducing liquid intake.

Since starting the macrobiotic diet, my overall condition has improved considerably, with only small setbacks. The twitching in my legs is now gone, and I need to use my stick less often than before. Also, the severe headaches from which I used to suffer have now gone away completely.

Type IV Hyperlipidemia

Peter Klein, M.D.

It was four years ago that I first heard about macrobiotics, after attending an introductory talk in Los Angeles. Following the lecture, most of us sat down to a macrobiotically prepared meal which began with *miso* soup and included grains and vegetables. I enjoyed the food and the company of the people I met. As I chewed my food, I began to think that this was something I should have started long ago. The meals got better and better as my sensitivity to taste improved, and I soon realized that I was doing something that could lead to a change in my health and well-being.

The idea of improving my health through natural methods had been evolving in me for quite a while, but the pressure and pace of my work and education, and especially of medical school, had left less and less time. However, in some ways I had come close to the macrobiotic diet. Once I had found it, though, I realized I was beginning a study that would involve unlearning as well as learning.

Eating macrobiotically has done a lot for me. It helped bring my cholesterol level down to normal and I now feel that the quality of my blood will continue to improve, along with the condition of my blood vessels and my condition in general. I no longer worry about the degeneration of blood vessels that plagued me when I found out that I had type IV hyperlipidemia.

The macrobiotic diet also helped lower my blood sugar level to normal; thus I stopped worrying about diabetes with its degeneration of the small arteries, "blindness," impotence, strokes, heart attacks, amputations, and nerve losses. Macrobiotics has also helped me with fears of gout, with its associated arthritis, possible kidney stones, and renal problems.

Since beginning to eat macrobiotically, I have had fewer colds, upper respiratory and throat infections, stomach upsets, and similar chronic problems, plus fewer conscious and unconscious fears about illness in general. This has been a great relief to me, since I have been plagued with illness from childhood, starting with an early reaction to cow's milk and the development of allergies, to severe asthma at the age of three. From then on I had difficulty in breathing and frequently stayed up all night until I discovered that if I rocked back and forth in bed, I would eventually pass out. However, I never knew if I would wake up or suffocate, and when I did wake up, I knew there would be another night of struggle.

After three episodes of severe upper respiratory infection, the last being a case of pneumonia, I was hospitalized and placed in an oxygen tent for several months. After this, I went to an asthmatic home in Denver. For the first time in life, I was free to play football, baseball, basketball, etc., and my condition improved. However, when I returned home, I occasionally had an attack until I moved to New Orleans to go to medical school.

While I was in medical school, my mother's doctor discovered that she had type IV hyperlipidemia and started her on Atronoid S. As soon as I found this out, I ran a test which showed that I also had type IV hyperlipedemia, along with a uric acid of 13.5 (normal is about 6). Hyperuricemia is usually a precursor of gout, and my elevated blood sugar (10) a possible precursor of diabetes. Afterward, my brother was tested and found to have a uric acid count of about 11. He decided to go on drug therapy. I decided I was not going to take any drugs, especially the one recommended for me, since I knew one out of a thousand people who took it developed leukemia, which is what my father had died from. I concluded that I must be putting something into my body that was causing me to have an abnormal chemistry, and decided to figure out how to get myself back in balance.

I decided to start by giving up animal foods, because their high protein content is converted to purine, which eventually shows up as uric acid. Animal foods such as dairy products and eggs are also high in the things that elevate the lipid level. I also started to eliminate sugar and sweets, since they often compromise the pancreas.

I had a lot to learn and, as a medical student, not much time to do it, especially since I had to work as many as thirty-nine hours a week to pay my way through medical school. However, even though I had some idea of the foods I had to give up, I did not know what to eat and how to prepare it. The medical literature on nutrition was of little help, since I could not find diets that excluded animal food and sugar, while the recommended substitutes were usually highly processed or synthetic foods.

During medical school I began to see more and more how the intake of certain substances contributed to illness and degeneration. It was easy to see how alcohol contributed to liver disease, pancreatitis and gastrointestinal problems, and how diets high in animal foods, dairy and eggs contributed to cardiovascular disease, as did obesity in general. It was also obvious that sugar could lead to the development of hypoglycemia and mild maturity onset diabetes, with related cardiovascular problems, heart attacks, strokes, blindness, impotence and amputations. I also saw how smoking and air pollution led to lung disease, and from my personal experience realized how milk and orange juice led to mucus deposits which contributed to difficulty in breathing and asthma. I also saw how stress and the rapid pace of life led to tension and possible hypertension, and how quick decisions based on poor judgment led to frequent accidents and mistakes.

As I became more observant of human behavior, it became obvious that many people had fixed patterns of thinking that prevented them from searching deeper and figuring out better and more enjoyable ways of doing things. During my internship in Los Angeles, I came to the conclusion that it would be much better to do whatever was necessary to prevent illness than to try and treat it once it developed. From working with many sick people, I saw how difficult it was to try to help them once their sickness had become acute. I had never worked so hard and seen so much tragedy, pain and frustration.

At some point I realized that hospitals and medicine were not going to provide the knowledge I was seeking, since they were concerned mostly with treating disease. After completing my internship, I started my psychiatry residency and took a job working at an emergency room on weekends. It was there that I treated an architect who introduced me to the East West Center in Los Angeles.

It was here that my exploration of macrobiotics began. It has been interesting, exciting, unique, perplexing and at times difficult, but I have continued to learn and my health has continued to improve. I have occasionally had reactions when I have decided to eat or try something that is not right for me. Whether I am aware of it or not, this disturbs the balance I am establishing, and thus I always learn from these experiences, eventually making the appropriate adjustments.

With that in mind I began to study individual and family development. I have frequently found that those who function best come from families that are physically, emotionally, intellectually and socially supportive, while appropriately setting beneficial limits that are not restrictive.

In order to help people make positive changes in their way of life, they need the same kind of support, encouragement and nurturance that a family and friends provide. I therefore use group therapy to help patients, with the group becoming a new pseudo-family which fosters beneficial development by providing an opportunity to share ideas on how to improve one's interactions with oneself, with others, and with the environment.

I would like to emphasize that you too can benefit from the support and encouragement of others who share your interest and desire for better health. Regular contact with them can facilitate emotional, intellectual and social well-being, along with physical improvement. Group activities such as dinners, discussions, group walks, exercises and others offer pleasant and enjoyable opportunities to share what you have done that has helped you.

For me, it is very enriching and rewarding to be involved in sharing with and helping others. My work is with the illnesses of greed, arrogance and disharmony that we have created and spread in this world. I would like to ask you to do what you can both for yourself and for others who need and will appreciate your help. It is from here that the proper understanding of how to create health will continue to spread to all who need and want it.

Macrobiotic Dietary Therapy in Japan

Hideo Ohmori
Tokyo, Japan

More than thirty years ago, at the end of World War II, Japan experienced the explosion of two atomic bombs, during which most of the people living in Hiroshima and Nagasaki died almost instantaneously. However, many of those who survived the immediate explosion later developed various forms of "atomic disease"—and have since died one by one.

At the time of the explosion, a man named Dr. Akizuki was directing the Department of Internal Medicine at St. Francis Hospital, located in Nagasaki near the center of the blast. Dr. Akizuki had been born with a natively small heart, which had been cured in a very short time by the macrobiotic way of eating. After this experience, he had decided to become a physician.

Prior to the explosion, he had been assigned to St. Francis Hospital where he was directing many people, at the same time continuing to study macrobiotics.

Immediately after the bomb exploded, he shouted to all of his staff and patients, "Take salt, take salt!" Of course, at that time, food shortages were very frequent in Japan, and as a result, the way of eating of most people was very simple: brown rice and *miso* soup containing a few vegetables, usually pumpkin or hard squash. The patients and hospital staff who were not under the direction of Dr. Akizuki died one by one as a result of the atomic explosion. However, Dr. Akizuki and the patients and staff in his department, all of whom were eating macrobiotically at that time, are all still alive and in very healthy condition.[2]

In Hiroshima, a fifty-year-old woman named Mrs. Taoka, who was macrobiotic, was living not too far from the center of the atomic blast. As a result of the explosion, fragments of shattered glass penetrated her entire body in about forty or fifty places. Also, her entire body was burned. She managed to escape from the city literally by crawling on the ground amidst what must have been tremendous confusion of destruction. When she began to search for brown rice, the farmers did not have any. However, she was able to obtain some barley, which she cooked with salt, and then also baked. After several days of eating cooked barley, she was able to get brown rice, and she began to eat a very good macrobiotic diet. However, during the following year, she experienced a continuous discharge of very black blood from her uterus. Gradually, as a result of her way of eating, healthy new blood started to form, and all of the pieces of glass which were deeply imbedded in her body naturally fell out, one by one. She is still alive, and is now in very extraordinary health.

---

[2] For further information, refer to *Macrobiotics, Cancer, and Medical Practice*, by Keith Block, M.D., in Chapter 2.

In Hiroshima, there was a high-school girl who was exposed to atomic radiation, and developed atomic disease. Her blood condition became bad, and as a result, she had been confined to bed for quite a while. She began macrobiotics not long afterward, and through dietary practice, cured her condition. She has since married, and is in very good health and now has seven children. Her husband is a professor at Hiroshima University, and they are both active in spreading the proper approach to macrobiotics among many of the citizens of Hiroshima through educational activities.

My experience in treating patients with macrobiotics began more than twenty years ago. During this time, I have met many cancer patients, and many of them have become better. About ten years ago, I was the director of a clinic which offered macrobiotic dietary treatment. Around that time, a young boy who had a very serious brain tumor was admitted. He was a student at Keio University and was examined at the University Hospital, which had given up on his case. At that time, he was paralyzed and trembling because of the tumor, and was carried into the clinic where he stayed for twenty days. For three years after that, I visited his home once a month. He has since completely overcome the tumor and is now married and has two children who are very happy and healthy.

A young boy who was scheduled to be operated on for stomach cancer at the Sapporo University Medical Center in Hokkaido escaped from the hospital and visited my home. He stayed there for three days during which I advised him to begin macrobiotics. After he left, I continued to advise him over the telephone. I visited America the following year, and upon my return to Japan, again went to Hokkaido for a series of lectures. I met him again there, and he was very happy since his condition had completely disappeared a long time ago. He is now active and busy.

At the present time in Japan, many cancers are being caused by the overconsumption of yin foods. For example, to illustrate, the atomic bomb dropped on Hiroshima left radioactive fall-out in the form of strontium 90, cobalt, cesium, etc. These elements create a yin influence since, according to spectroscopic analysis, they evidence a more purplish or bluish color, which is more yin. Salt, however, has the opposite tendency. According to spectroscopic analysis, the sodium in salt gives off a more orange or red color, which is more yang. It was for this reason, to offset the effects of radiation, that Dr. Akizuki recommended that his staff and patients take salt. Since many cancers in Japan are the result of yin, when we approach this problem, we try to control the intake of yin foods, such as sugar, milk, cold drinks, fruit juice, soft drinks, chemicals, etc.

According to our experience, if cancer is still in the beginning or middle stages, it can easily be cured by food alone, without any particular external application. However, in more advanced cases, it is often necessary to use external applications together with the practice of good diet. A typical treatment for many cases is a plaster made with taro potato. When applied to the skin, this application helps to absorb, or pull out, various cancer toxins toward and then out through the skin.

For example, in the case of a person who suffers from stomach cancer resulting from the excessive intake of sugar, if we apply this taro potato plaster, then a black almost charcoal-like tar will start to appear on the skin. In my experience, tumors the size of a fist have disappeared in one month from the correct application of this plaster.

I have found that the cause of a particular cancer can often be determined by its location. Generally speaking, cancers which appear in the compacted organs, such as the kidneys, liver, or pancreas, are usually caused by too much yang food in the form of eggs, meat, and other animal products. On the other hand, when cancer appears in the more hollow, expanded organs, like the stomach or intestines, it is generally caused by more yin; that is, fruit juice, sugar, chemicals, etc. Also, cancer can appear in either the upper or lower portion of the body, and again, the cause is slightly different in each case. For example, cancer of the prostate is caused generally by too much animal food. To offset this, our dietary approach should include a reduction in the intake of salt, and the elimination of animal food.

Of course, for each individual case, we also need to adjust the ratio of main food, or whole grain cereals, to supplemental food. Recently for patients in Japan who have developed cancer because of too much animal food, I have been recommending barley as the principal grain, rather than brown rice. Of course, our overall recommendations should vary with each person's age, sex, and condition.

The differences in the types of cancer prevalent in Japan and in the United States are primarily the result of the different dietary habits of each country. At the present time, Japanese people are eating large quantities of refined white rice, while vegetables, which form their main supplemental food, are often cooked in sugar. This type of food remains in the stomach for a longer than normal period of time.

In America, sugar is usually taken in a more liquid form, such as in coffee, soft drinks, etc. Compared with most people in America, most people in Japan do not eat as much meat. However, refined white rice is very soft, and can therefore be swallowed without much chewing, resulting in a more acidic condition in the stomach.

Even though the consumption of sugar may be less in Japan than in the United States, by eating such a consistently large volume of refined rice, Japanese people tend to develop more stomach cancer. In the United States, people are eating what I consider to be an excessive quantity of animal food, which often results in a weakening of the intestinal condition, in many cases leading to the development of colon and other intestinal cancers. However, the consumption of meat and other animal products is increasing in both countries, and I feel that both countries will experience a corresponding increase in the incidence of colon and other intestinal cancers.

With a diet consisting of 100 percent animal food, such as that eaten by the Eskimos, cancer rarely develops. At the same time, in people who live near the equator, in a very hot tropical climate, and who eat the native diet consisting of mostly vegetables and fruits, cancer is very rare. For example, the people who were living around the area where Dr. Albert Schweitzer had his clinic, were eating large quantities of bananas, and instead of cancer, a more prevalent sickness was leprosy. Cancer develops more in advanced, modernized societies, especially where excessive amounts of animal products and sugar are consumed. Cancer often seems to result from the combined effects of meat and other types of yang animal foods, with sugar and other types of yin food.

Before World War II, cancer was the nineteenth leading cause of death in Japan. Since the war, however, food patterns have changed enormously with the consumption of meat and other animal products and the consumption of sugar increasing tremendously every year. At the same time, the increase in the number of deaths caused by cancer has consistently paralleled the increase in the consumption of these foods, so that, in 1972, cancer became the second leading cause of death. Since the consumption of these foods continues to increase day by day, I feel we can also expect a corresponding increase in the incidence of cancer.

Macrobiotic Dietary Therapy in Veterinary Practice

Norman Ralston, D.V.M.
Dallas, Texas

In our veterinary practice in Texas, we have observed that a yin condition generally seems to prevail in dogs today. We believe this condition is initially due to the high water content in most canned dog food and/or the cooking and processing methods used to cause expansion in most commercial dog foods. In both cases, a yin, expanded condition in the food is created, and passed on to the dog.

This condition is worsened when an already yin dog ingests the mixture of metabolic waste and hydrogenated fats found in these commercially prepared pet foods. Hydrogenated fats are processed animal fats that the dog appears instinctively to reject. The body stores these materials in less active places (like fat pons on the hips), or it discharges them. The food also contains strong chemicals the body recognizes as foreign and unnatural, and therefore tries to expel.

We see these discharges through the eyes and nose, vagina, and in the form of waxy stools, as the body fights to survive the onslaught of unnatural substances. At the same time, the body is suffering from lack of wholesome nutrition and the olfactory nerves and taste buds are stimulated artificially. The animal therefore eats more, creating more of an overload on the body's excretory system, until finally there is a breakdown. There is only one thing left for the body to do at this point: stop taking in nourishment altogether. We often recognize this syndrome when an owner brings in an animal that refuses to eat.

If given a chance, the body will free itself of these detrimental substances. A fast of about three days will accomplish this. Within a natural environment a fast occurs when an animal fails to kill its prey for a period of days. When such natural fasts do not occur, and the body is continually presented with more and more of these substances that it recognizes as foreign or toxic, this excess is stored in more and more places, eventually resulting in a toxemia condition that may not at first be clinically recognized.

These unnatural substances are destroying our pet population. We see this manifesting through all kinds of degenerative diseases, from cancer to cataracts. Still more important, we are seeing weaker and weaker litters of puppies being born.

An amazing transformation can be seen if we simply put the animal on a diet of freshly cooked whole grain, a little rare cooked meat, and whatever (cooked) fresh vegetables are available locally, excluding the more yin varieties.

We have repeatedly used this approach to diet at our clinic. We feel the most important part of our treatment is the dietary change. We vary this according to the situation; when we find large nodular growths in the breasts of females, for example, we withhold fats of any kind, even vegetable fats. We substitute beans for the meat portion of the diet, so that the body will be fat-starved and literally feed on itself. This seems to help.

Rather than classifying a growth as "malignant" or "nonmalignant," we view the presence of *any* growth as an expression from the body that it is trying to rid itself of something. We stay away from surgery, at least initially. Experience with ginger compress and albi plaster[3] on my own body have inspired me to try it on conditions warranting its use in animals.

If the growth is located where it can be bandaged readily, we apply an albi plaster after cleaning up the area, and usually leave it on overnight. These plasters are repeated daily; but we play this part by ear, having the owner apply them at home as much as possible. If the growth has shrunk and we can feel that it is fairly free from the body, we may make a small skin incision and take it out. We do this especially if we feel that the owner is tired of treating the animal and is likely to take it to another vet to have it put to sleep. After surgical removal of the growth, we again apply the albi plaster. We want the body to remember which way we want the growth to go: off the body. The following case is typical of our general approach:

In 1978, a thirteen-year-old mixed chihuahua was presented with typical signs of congestive heart failure, as previously diagnosed. The animal was presently taking digitalis and a diuretic called lasix, was cyanotic, temperature 100°F; respiratory rate could be noted without the use of a stethoscope. The owner reported that the animal coughed with almost every breath. Due to the gravity of the situation, the animal was handled with caution for fear she would die on the examination table. The animal also had early cataracts.

Because of the expanded heart and obesity of the animal, we could say this was a yin disease. In addition to diet, we needed to use some treatment that would help rapidly discharge this excessive yin (particularly from about the eyes, heart and lungs) and allow the animal's condition to contract. Grated ginger root and taro potato plaster seemed to fit the description, so we decided to try it.

Using an ordinary kotex pad on which we placed grated ginger, we taped the kotex pad with the ginger next to the skin just above the eyes using elasti-kon tape. The tape was applied loosely and great care was exercised to see that the breathing was in no way hindered. We felt it would be better to let the animal get the bandage off rather than kill herself trying.

Then, using a disposable diaper, a poultice of grated taro potato was applied over the entire ventral surface of the chest cavity. A body stockinette was applied to hold the poultice in place. Elastikon was applied to the stockinette to anchor it in place, and the poultices were left in place overnight.

On the following morning, I was pleasantly surprised to find most of the

---

[3] See Appendix, Chapter 1.

fluid gone from the chest cavity. The animal was more alert with a pink tongue and breathing was easier. The heartbeat was regular and the overall condition seemed better. The treatment was repeated by just rolling the stockinette back and changing the diaper with new grated potato added.

The animal was sent home with the following instructions. The animal was to receive the following diet and nothing more: 50 percent whole grain brown rice, 25 percent lean hamburger meat cooked by boiling, and 25 percent steamed vegetables. To this we added 1/8 teaspoon of sea meal (ground seaweed) daily.

The animal has continued to show improvement and has undergone anesthesia with ketaset and acepromazine to have her teeth cleaned.

Following the tradition of self-criticism, I would say the case is not complete because we should have had before and after x-rays to confirm the diagnosis of right heart enlargement. However, under the circumstances, I feel justified in not taking them. The stress of holding the animal for her x-ray could have resulted in her death.

We realize our limited number of cases, along with the lack of biopsy reports, leaves this work open to question. However, to yield to the temptation to get a confirmed diagnosis or a name we can call the growth, would be defeating our purpose. It would, in effect, be putting the cart before the horse. Consider the Oriental view of the seven levels of health care: diet and daily activity are considered number one, and surgery number seven. By doing a biopsy, we would in effect be putting surgery number one.

Food Policy Recommendations for the United States

Michio Kushi

In the United States, as well as in other modern nations over the past few decades, people have been experiencing the effects of the biological and sociological degeneration of humanity. The tendency toward this degeneration includes the following aspects:
1. Increase of chronic diseases among people in all walks of life.
2. Increase of mental and psychological disorders among people in all walks of life.
3. Increase of uncontrollable behavior, especially among children and the younger generation.
4. Increase in the abuse of hallucinogenic drugs.
5. Decline in the working efficiency of people at all levels of employment, and increasing loss of work time due to illness.
6. Decline in the spirit of respect for traditional values and the older generation as well as a decline in direct love for children and the younger generation.
7. Increasing decomposition of harmonious family unity.
8. Increase in the crime rate including violent crimes, especially among younger people.

If this tendency continues to accelerate at its present rate for another two decades, American society will face serious impairment of its economic, political, social, religious, educational and cultural vitality.

Having examined this physical, mental and social trend for over twenty years, we have come to the conclusion that the major cause of this general phenomenon lies in what the majority of individuals and families consume daily through their present dietary practice.

Accordingly, we have devoted ourselves, for the past twenty years, to educational activities to promote a better understanding of quality food, including its production, processing, preparation and consumption. Our educational activities, involving lectures, seminars, publications and personal contact, have contributed to promoting a trend toward the natural food movement in the United States as well as several countries in Europe.

As a whole, those people who have practiced our dietary recommendations have recovered for themselves a more healthy and sound life, regaining physical, mental and spiritual balance, as well as developing more efficient study and work habits. For documentation, please see the case history reports published by the East West Foundation. The cases reported include recovery from the following problems:
1. Cancer, arthritis, epilepsy, heart disease, skin diseases, chronic digestive troubles, general fatigue and other physical problems.
2. Mental fatigue, depression, anxiety, fear and other psychological disorders.
3. Misunderstanding and quarreling within families, including aspects of the so-called generation gap.
4. Disrespect for the traditional values and spirit of hard-working ancestors.

5. Chaotic and disorderly life-styles.
6. Abuse of hallucinogenic drugs.

Our Food Policy Recommendations

We would recommend the following general points:

(1) In order to preserve the natural, health building qualities of food, there should be no, or at least fewer, chemicals used in the production and processing of food. The current overrefined and other extremely artificial treatment of foods should be gradually reduced as much as possible.

(2) Agriculture should gradually shift from the current style of artificial mass production to a more natural style of production, in order to restore quality.

(3) Food preparation should become more home-style, reemphasizing the kitchen of every home as the site for most cooking rather than mass preparation, particularly in the current highly commercial, "pre-packaged" and "fast food" style.

(4) Food for daily consumption should consist of two basic categories: principal food and supplementary food.

   a) The principal staple to be unrefined whole cereal grains and their products. They should constitute approximately 50 percent or more of the daily intake. Examples of such foods are: whole wheat, brown rice, oats, barley, rye, millet, corn, and buckwheat, in all their varieties such as bread, pasta, etc.

   b) The supplementary food to include several categories which should vary according to regional and seasonal environmental conditions as well as personal needs. Examples of such foods are: vegetables, beans, sea vegetables, fruits, seeds and nuts, fish and other seafood, poultry and eggs (in occasion).

In general, artificial beverages and highly aromatic stimulant foods and drinks are not recommended for daily consumption. The current heavy reliance on meat, mass-produced, non-fertilized eggs and highly refined or industrially treated food products and drinks is also to be discouraged. Such foods should be recommended only if they have been processed in a way that keeps the natural quality through traditional methods. Reliance on sugar and similar mono- and disaccharide sweeteners should be replaced by shifting to polysaccharide sweets, mainly processed from grains and vegetables.

(5) In addition to food composition, proper selection of quality food and proper cooking of these foods is also important. We recommend sea salt for cooking instead of highly refined, mined salt, and cold-pressed, pure quality vegetable oil instead of chemically and high-temperature processed oil. For seasoning and to aid digestion of grains, we recommend traditional foods such as pickled vegetables and naturally fermented soybean products (such as soy sauce, *miso*, *tempeh*, etc.).

(6) We recommend the traditional custom of families cooking and eating together at least once a day, in order to assure each family's health and to strengthen mutual understanding among family members as well as family friends.

(7) The cost of food for the recommended diet becomes approximately one-third the cost of present dietary practice even though all daily nutritional requirements are met as well as and in fact, much more easily than by the present American diet. This saving alone could be of great help in recovering a sound economical condition for individual families and society as a whole.

National Benefits

If the United States reorients its food goals in a direction similar to that proposed here, aspects of various social problems would eventually be reduced considerably. The benefits resulting from such a policy would include the following areas:

(1) The general health of the American public will become much sounder. This improvement could save enormous amounts of money at every level from family, community, city and state to federal. Expenditures saved on health care could be used for more productive and creative uses.

(2) Schools and other educational facilities can function much more smoothly as a result of the native emotional and intellectual balance which students and teachers will naturally recover.

(3) The rate of crimes, including violent acts, will decrease substantially, resulting in a much safer, less fear-ridden and more peaceful society, as well as saving large amounts of money currently spent on police and legal procedures.

(4) Divorce and breakup of families, as well as general conflicts in human relations, will decrease significantly. Natural, caring relationships will eventually be restored throughout the society, leading to happier personal and community life as a whole. This easing of current tensions between individuals and economic racial groups will reduce the present need for governmental regulatory control of the people.

(5) All private enterprises, companies, institutions and public organizations will benefit from the increased efficiency that comes from the recovery of sound physical and mental health in people. This change will ensure the destiny of the country toward a far greater prosperity.

(6) The population the country is able to support comfortably will be substantially increased as a result of switching to consumption of grains and beans by human beings rather than the current indirect consumption of these foods in the form of meat.

Programs Recommended

There are, of course, enormous problems which will have to be solved in order to achieve the goal of the above recommendations. It cannot be expected that the above recommendations could be put into practice in a short period of time. We estimate that it will take approximately twenty years before the majority of the United States can shift in this general direction. In the meantime, all our efforts, public and personal, should be directed to the following concerns:

(1) The reorientation of government agencies toward a new policy on food and agriculture should be designed within a reasonably short period of time.

(2) A program of education for food producers including farmers, processors and manufacturers should be designed with the goal of producing better, more natural, food, if possible, with the assistance of Federal, state and local government. Conventions, conferences, seminars, publications and the media should be involved in these educational programs.

(3) Schools, hospitals, hotels, restaurants, airlines and other public eating places should be educated in the use of better quality food and better application of cooking methods avoiding as much as possible synthetic chemicalized and overly refined foods and beverages. Such education can also be promoted through conferences, conventions, lectures, discussions and publication of guidebooks.

(4) Families, as well as individuals, should be educated about good food. Such edu-

cation could be spread through lectures, conferences and discussions with women's associations, community organizations, and social clubs as well as adult education. Magazines, newspapers, television and other media should also be asked to participate.

(5) In this connection, establishing a public educational team for community health resembling the "Peace Corps" might be considered. The education and training of such community workers may take six months to one year before they begin their actual educational services in society. Education for the members of a community health service should include:

a) General theories of nutrition, modern and traditional, and the relationship of diet to major physical and mental disorders.

b) Difference in the technique and results of organic, nonchemicalized agriculture as compared with artificial, energy-intensive agriculture, including field visits.

c) Practical study of food selection and cooking until the participants are qualified to guide individuals and families. Some members should also become capable of guiding the cooking in public eating places such as restaurants and hotels, as well as institutional eating places.

d) Study of practical methods of simple food processing such as baking, pickling, etc. for home use.

e) Understanding of rules and regulations related to foods and beverages.

f) Learning practical family counseling.

(6) Medical practitioners also should be encouraged to recommend proper food to patients as part of therapy. Education of medical professionals is recommended in the relationship between food and disease. Such education can be included in the educational programs of medical schools as well as by the establishment of alternative medical schools, plus lectures, seminars, discussions and conferences for medical people.

Conclusion

A shift from the present dietary trends in the United States to a more sound practice will result in improved economic welfare for the country. A sizeable portion of the agricultural products of the nation, including grains, beans and sea vegetables, can be exported to other countries which presently suffer from general malnutrition. This policy will also reduce general costs of living and public expenditures, substantially lower food costs, medical expenses, Social Security and Welfare expenses and will improve general working efficiency. It can be foreseen that our country will develop in this way toward a healthy, peaceful, intellectual, happier and more prosperous future.

However, this shift should be neither radical nor unreasonably fast. It should proceed in gradual steps within every community and industry as producers, suppliers and consumers are able to adapt. Accordingly, educational services for the above described area should be conducted very actively.

Supplement

Study and research on the following subjects under the encouragement of Federal, state, and local government are to be considered:

1. Study on the expected change in social and economic patterns throughout the country as present dietary practice is shifted toward a new, but more traditional, dietary practice: this study should possibly include the influence of various social

and economic changes over periods of the next five, ten, fifteen, twenty and twenty-five years.

2. Study on the possible change in economic function of social groups on all levels from the family, through communities and institutions, up to the governmental level of expenditures, as the above changes in dietary patterns take place.

3. Research on the use of more natural, non-chemical fertilization processes in agriculture and research on the collecting methods of agriculture which were practiced throughout the world until the early part of this century, especially in Asian countries where labor intensive methods have been particularly developed. This research should study the feasibility of gradually shifting to natural, non-chemical fertilization applied to large scale agricultural production.

4. Research on expected changes in food cost, including cost of production and price for the consumer, in the event agricultural production is gradually shifted from reliance on chemical fertilizers, herbicides and pesticides to more natural methods.

5. Research on the technology of traditional food processing, still preserved in some areas of the world, including methods for processing grains, beans, vegetables and fruits. This research should include study of methods of traditional fermentation as used, for example, in producing *miso* and soy sauce, as well as other fermented foods including pickled vegetables.

6. Research on methods of collecting and using various sea plants, sea vegetables and moss for inclusion as supplements to daily food consumption.

7. Research on methods of processing vegetable oils, comparing current techniques of high-temperature, chemical processing with low-temperature, non-chemical processing; such research should study the differences between the two with respect to qualities and effects on human health as well as cost of production.

8. Research on the effects on human health of refined disaccharides and monosaccharides such as white sugar, as compared with the use of unrefined complex sugars, or polysaccharides. This research should include a study of the economic factors involved in a gradual shift from the use of refined sugar and honey to the use of grain and other complex sugars.

9. Research on the effect on human health of the current abundant use of dairy food and studies on the effects of reducing the use of it, including its replacement by unsaturated fats of vegetable origin, such as sesame butter and bean-based milk (e.g. *tofu*).

10. Research on reduced need for vitamin supplements in the event that more natural, unrefined foods become widely used in daily consumption.

11. Research on the effect on human health of the current large use of tropical and semi-tropical products including fruits, fruit juices and spices growing in climates differing from that of the United States, compared with the use of fruits, fruit juices and seasonings indigenous to this country.

12. Research on the effect on human health of the current large consumption of soft drinks and artificial beverages compared with the effects on human health of more natural and traditional beverages.

13. Study of the possibility of including courses in health, food and cooking in the upper grades of elementary schools and/or during certain years at the high school level.

14. Research on the difference in the effect on human health between highly refined salt and traditionally processed sea salt.

15. Research on the influence of environmental factors, including the quality of air and water, on agricultural products and human health, especially in crowded cities and industrial areas.

As initial steps, the following programs are recommended for application as soon as possible.

1. Clear indication of the contents and additivies in the labeling of every food product and beverage.
2. Such clear indication of contents and additivies may be enlarged in its application not only to products on the market but also to foods on the menus of public eating places.
3. Health education related to food should be encouraged in all public schools and educational institutions.
4. Medical schools should be strongly encouraged to increase the number of courses available on food and its relation to health. Also, an educational institution for medicine dealing widely with problems of health, from a holistic view of environmental conditions, should be established.

East West Foundation — Diet and Health Related Activities, 1972-1982

• *1972–73.*   Participation with a research team from the Harvard Medical School in Boston, led by Frank Sacks, M.D. and associates, in conducting a series of studies on the effects of macrobiotic dietary patterns on blood pressure and cholesterol levels. These studies demonstrated that the macrobiotic dietary approach can significantly reduce two of the leading risk factors in the development of cardiovascular illnesses, currently the leading causes of death in the United States and many other industrialized countries. (See reports on these and subsequent research projects in Chapter 3.)

• *1974–75.*   Coordination of Michio Kushi Seminars on the "Principles and Practice of Oriental Medicine" in Boston and New York. More than thirty seminars were presented, including introductory, intermediate, and advanced level studies. Over five-hundred doctors, chiropractors, and health professionals participated in these seminars, which introduced the theory and practice of acupuncture, dietary adjustment, and related health approaches.

• *1975.*   Arrangement and coordination of the first Michio Kushi Seminar in London, in association with the East West Center and British Acupuncture Association. A full week of seminars on the "Principles and Practice of Oriental Medicine" were presented at the London Tara Hotel, and attended by more than two-hundred doctors and health professionals. This event was followed by a seminar in Paris, and by ongoing Kushi International Seminars throughout Western Europe, South America, and the Far East. Thousands of people, including many health professionals, have participated in these events.

• Presentation of the first summer residential program on "Oriental Medicine, Philosophy, and Culture" at Amherst College in Amherst, Massachusetts. Seven residential programs were presented at Amherst College and Pine Manor College between 1975 and 1981.

• Coordination and presentation of the "Integral Medicine Program" in association with the Department of Continuing Education at the University of Massachusetts at Amherst. More than two-hundred students from the five-college Amherst area participated in this program.

• Presentation of the first "Natural Food Symposium" at Boston University. Speakers included Michio Kushi and Francis Moore Lappé, author of *Diet for a Small Planet*. Over one-thousand people attended.

• Compilation and publication of the first *Case History Report*, which included personal accounts of the recovery from numerous disorders through macrobiotics. Seven issues of the *Case History Report* were published and distributed from 1975–1980.

• *1976.*   Publication and distribution of *A Dietary Approach to Cancer According to the Principles of Macrobiotics*, which included material from Mr. Kushi's lectures together with a preliminary presentation of cancer related case histories. This report was sent to over two-hundred international cancer research centers and health organizations including the National Cancer Institute, the American Health Foundation, the World Health Organization, and others, and was distributed to the general public.

• *1977.*   Presentation of the first conference on "A Nutritional Approach to Cancer" at

Pine Manor College in Chestnut Hill, Massachusetts, for the purpose of reviewing current evidence on the relationship of diet to degenerative disorders, and to discuss possible avenues for further communication in this area. Conference participants included Michio Kushi, Robert S. Mendelsohn, M.D., Stephen Appelbaum, Ph.D., of the Menninger Foundation, Richard Prindle, M.D. formerly of the World Health Organization, Frank Spiezer, M.D. of the Harvard Medical School, Hideo Ohmori of the Japan Macrobiotic Association, and others. The proceedings of this conference were later published and again distributed to the appropriate agencies, as well as to the general public.

• Presentation of the "World Without Cancer Symposium" at Boston University. Speakers included Michio Kushi, William Dufty, author of *Sugar Blues*, and Gloria Swanson. Over six-hundred people attended.

• *1977–78.* Arrangement of several White House meetings at which Mr. Kushi's *Food Policy Recommendations for the United States* were presented (see preceding Appendix); presentation by Mr. Kushi of a special address at the United Nations on "One Peaceful World through Macrobiotics."

• *1978.* Publication and distribution of the *Macrobiotic Way of Natural Healing* (currently titled *Natural Healing through Macrobiotics*) by Michio Kushi, edited by Edward Esko and Marc Van Cauwenberghe, M.D., with a foreword by Robert S. Mendelsohn, M.D.

• Arrangement and coordination of meetings between Mr. Kushi (and associates) and leading individuals in the nutrition and health field, including Dr. Mark Hegsted, formerly of the Harvard School of Public Health, Dr. Phillip Lee, of the University of California, Gio B. Gori, Ph.D., formerly of the National Cancer Institute, and Nicholas Mottern and Chris Hitt, formerly of the Senate Select Committee on Nutrition and Human Needs.

• Presentation of the second annual conference on a "Nutritional Approach to Cancer and Degenerative Disorders" at Amherst College. Participants in the conference included Michio Kushi, Robert S. Mendelsohn, M.D., Edward Kass, M.D. and Frank Sacks, M.D., both of the Harvard Medical School, Mrs. Marilyn Light, President of the American Hypoglycemia Association, Mrs. Marion Tompson, President of the La Leche League, International, William Dufty, Nicholas Mottern, principal author of *Dietary Goals for the United States* (released the previous year), William Tara, and as a special guest, Mrs. Lima Ohsawa of the Japan Macrobiotic Association.

• Formation of the East West Foundation Medical/Scientific Advisory Board with a number of conference participants, to assist in the coordination and supervision of future programs in this field.

• Participation with Jean and Mary Alice Kohler of Muncie, Indiana, in the preparation and publication of their book, *Healing Miracles from Macrobiotics* (see Bibliography). In February, 1980, shortly after the appearance of this book, Mr. Kohler appeared in a nationwide fifty-city broadcast of public interest in the macrobiotic approach. By popular demand, the show was repeated in August, 1980.

• *1979.* Presentation of the third annual conference on a "Nutritional Approach to Cancer and Degenerative Disorders" in Boston. The third conference was attended by many of the participants from preceding conferences, and also included special presentations by Anthony J. Sattilaro, M.D., President of the Methodist Hospital in Philadelphia, Norman Ralston, D.V.M., and Chandras Thakkur, M.D., an authority on traditional Indian medicine, from Bombay.

• *1980.* Compilation and publication of the first edition of *Cancer and Diet* for distribution to various international health and research agencies and to the general public.

• Presentation of regular "Cancer and Diet" seminars in the Boston area. During the following year, these seminars were presented in various North American cities, in cooperation with the North American Macrobiotic Congress.

• Presentation of the fourth annual conference on a "Nutritional Approach to Cancer and Degenerative Disorders" in Boston. This event was attended by many of the participants from previous conferences, and featured presentations by Keith Block, M.D., Peter Klein, M.D., Christiane Northrup, M.D., and Michael Jacobson, of the Center for Science and the Public Interest in Washington, D.C.

• *1980–81.* Preparation and distribution of over 40,000 direct mail packets regarding macrobiotics, in response to publicity such as the publication of "An M.D. Heals Himself of Cancer" by Anthony J. Sattilaro, M.D. and Tom Monte, in the *East West Journal*, the *Saturday Evening Post* (September, 1980), the *Denver Post*, and other newspapers throughout the country.

• Publication and distribution of a second, revised edition of *Cancer and Diet*, which included material from previous conferences and "Cancer and Diet" seminars.

• Introduction of the Macrobiotic Lunch Program at the Lemuel Shattuck Hospital in Boston, in cooperation with Paul Schulman, former Director of the Shattuck Hospital, and the Kushi Foundation.

• *1981.* Presentation of an active "Macrobiotic Community Education" program in the Boston area, including radio and television appearances; free lectures at Public Libraries; presentations at hospitals, nursing associations, and women's groups; and classes at natural food stores throughout New England.

• Presentation of a symposium, "Your Diet, Your Health: Preventive Medicine in the 80s," at Boston University. Speakers included Michio Kushi, William Castelli, M.D., Christiane Northrup, M.D., Richard Donze, D.O., and William Dufty. More than six-hundred people attended.

• Presentation of a symposium on "Macrobiotics and Preventive Health Care" at Boston University, followed by the fifth annual conference on a "Nutritional Approach to Cancer and Degenerative Disorders." Special presentations were made by William Castelli, M.D., Michio Kushi, William Dufty, Keith Block, M.D., Frank Kern, Frank Sacks, M.D., Peter Klein, M.D., Donald Wong-Ken, D.O., of the Waterville Osteopathic Hospital in Waterville, Maine, Blaine Friedlander, of the Forensic Habilitation Institute in Fairfax, Virginia, and others.

• Presentation of a conference at the Forensic Habilitation Institute in Fairfax, Virginia, to discuss the possibility of implementing macrobiotic food programs in corrections and mental health facilities.

• *1981–82.* Publication and distribution of the *Cancer Prevention Diet*. This book included a special section on Diet and Heart Disease, and was distributed to many medical professionals and health practitioners, as well as to the general public.

• Coordination, together with the Kushi Institute, of the Macrobiotic Cook Referral Service, which offers trained macrobiotic cooks for institutional and home service.

Bibliography

Aihara, Cornellia. *Macrobiotic Kitchen: Key to Good Health*. Tokyo: Japan Publications, Inc. *The Dō of Cooking*. 4 vols., Oroville, Calif.: George Ohsawa Macrobiotic Foundation.

"An M.D. Who Conquered His Cancer," *Saturday Evening Post*. Indianapolis, Ind.: 1980.

Ardell, Donald B. *High Level Wellness*. Bantam, 1979

Bergan JG. and Brown PT. "Nutritional Status of 'New' Vegetarians." *Journal of the American Dietetic Association*, 76(2): 151–155, 1980.

Cancer: A Manual for Practitioners. 5th ed., American Cancer Society, 1978.

Clinical Oncology for Medical Students and Physicians, 5th ed., the University of Rochester School of Medicine: the American Cancer Society, 1978.

Cousins, Norman. *Anatomy of an Illness as Perceived by the Patient*. 1979.

Dufty, William. *Sugar Blues*. New York: Warner Publications.

East West Foundation. *Cancer and Diet*. Brookline, Mass.: East West Publications, 1980.

East West Foundation. *The Cancer Prevention Diet*. Ibid., 1981.

East West Foundation. *The Macrobiotic Approach to Cancer*. Ibid., 1982.

East West Journal. Monthly. Ibid.

Esko, Wendy. *Introducing Macrobiotic Cooking*. Tokyo: Japan Publications, Inc.

Esko, Edward and Wendy. *Macrobiotic Cooking for Everyone*. Ibid.

Knuiman JT and West CE. "The Concentration of Cholesterol in Serum and in Various Lipoproteins in Macrobiotic, Vegetarian, and Non-vegetarian Men and Boys." *Atherosclerosis*.

Kohler, Jean and Mary Alice. *Healing Miracles From Macrobiotics*. Englewood Cliffs, N.J.: Parker Publishing Co.

Kushi Institute Study Guide. Bi–monthly. Brookline, Mass.: Kushi Institute.

Kushi, Aveline. *How to Cook with Miso*. Tokyo: Japan Publications, Inc.

Kushi, Michio. *The Book of Dō-In*. Ibid.

Kushi, Michio. *The Book of Macrobiotics*. Ibid.

Kushi, Michio. *How to See Your Health: The Book of Oriental Diagnosis*. Ibid.

Kushi Micho. *Macrobiotic Dietary Recommendations*. Brookline, Mass.: East West Foundation.

Kushi Michio. *Macrobiotics: Experience the Miracle of Life*. Ibid.

Kushi, Michio. *Natural Healing through Macrobiotics*. Tokyo: Japan Publications, Inc.

Kushi, Michio. *Oriental Diagnosis*. London: Sunwheel Publications.

Kushi, Michio. *Visions of a New World: The Era of Humanity*. Brookline, Mass: East West Journal.

LeShan, Lawrence, Ph.D. *You Can Fight For Your Life*. Jove Publications Inc., 1978.

Macrobiotic Case Histories. 7 Vols., Brookline, Mass.: East West Foundation.

Macrobiotic Review. Quarterly. Baltimore, Md.: East West Foundation.

Mendelsohn, Robert S. *Confession of A Medical Heretic*. Chicago, Ill.: Contemporary Books.

Mendelsohn, Robert S. *Male Practice*. Ibid.

Monte T. "The Staff of Life." *East West Journal. 10*(11): 47, 1980.

Ohsawa, George. *The Book of Judgement*. Oroville, Calif.: George Ohsawa Macrobiotic Foundation.

Ohsawa, George. *Cancer and the Philosophy of the Far East*. Binghamton, N.Y.: Swan House.

Ohsawa, George. *Guidebook for Living*. Oroville, Calif.: George Ohsawa Macrobiotic Foundation.

Ohsawa, George, *Zen Macrobiotics*. Ibid.

Ohsawa, Lima. *The Art of Just Cooking*. Brookline, Mass.: Autumn Press.

Order of the Universe. Quarterly. Brookline, Mass.: Kushi Institute.

Pelletier, Kenneth. *Holistic Medicine, from Stress to Optium Health*. 1979.

A Physician's Handbook on Orthomolecular Medicine. Edited by Roger Williams, Ph.D., Pergamon, 1977.

Sacks FM, Donner A, Castelli WP, et al. "Effect of Ingestion of Meat on Plasma Cholesterol of Vegetarians." *Journal of the American Medical Association. 246*(6): 640–644, 1981.

Sacks FM, Castelli WP, and Kass EH. "Plasma Lipids and Lipoproteins in Vegetarians and Controls." *New England Journal of Medicine*. Boston, Mass.: 1975.

Sacks FM, Rosner B and Kass EH. "Blood Pressure in Vegetarians." *American Journal of Epidemiology*. Vol. 100, No. 5. Baltimore, Md.: John Hopkins University, 1974.

Sattilaro, Anthony J. and Monte, Tom. *Recalled by Life; The Story of a Recovery from Cancer*. Boston: Houghton-Mifflin, 1982.

Selye, Hans. *Stress Without Distress*. Lippincott, 1974.

Shealy, C. Norman. *90 Days to Self-Health*. Dial, 1977.

Simonton, O. Carl, Matthews-Simonton, Spehanie, Creighton, James.*Getting Well Again*. 1978.

United States Senate Select Committee on Nutrition and Human Needs. *Dietary Goals for the United States*. Washington, D.C.: U.S. Government Printing Office, 1977.

Whelan, Elizabeth, Ph.D. *Preventing Cancer*. Norton, 1978.

Yamamoto, Shizuko. *Barefoot Shiatsu*. Tokyo: Japan Publications, Inc.

Notes on the Contributors

Keith Block M.D., Ph. D. received his Bachelor of Science degree from the University of Florida and University of London in 1975. He graduated from the University of Miami School of Medicine in 1979, and participated in a Medical Residency Program at the Illinois Masonic Medical Center. He has done post-doctoral work on immunization/infectious disease/and nutrition, and is practicing privately in Evanston, Illinois, where he incorporates nutritional approaches in the care of a variety of conditions. He has been practicing the macrobiotic way of life since 1975, and is currently the Medical/Nutritional Consultant for CBS Radio in Chicago. Dr. Block is completing two books on the subjects of a controversial look into vaccination practice and a macrobiotic primer. He is a regular columnist for the *East West Jounal* and lectures throughout the United States.

Richard Donze, D.O. received his undergraduate degree from the University of Pennsylvania, and his medical degree from the Philadelphia College of Osteopathic Medicine. He is presently integrating advice on diet and life-style with family medicine at the Family Medicine Clinic at the Methodist Hospital in Philadelphia.

William Castelli, M.D. graduated from Yale in 1953, and received his medical degree at the University of Louraine in Belgium in 1959. He conducted his internship at the Kings County Hospital Center in Brooklyn, New York, and his residency at the Lemuel Shattuck Hospital in Boston. From 1962–65, he completed a post-doctoral fellowship in Preventive Medicine at Harvard, and joined the Framingham Heart Study in 1965. Dr. Castelli currently lectures on Preventive Medicine and Epidemiology at the Harvard Medical School, and is an adjunct Associate Professor at the Boston University School of Medicine. He is also a lecturer in medicine at the University of Massachusetts Medical School in Worcester, and has authored more than 50 publications dealing with the natural history of coronary disease.

Edward Esko began the study of macrobiotics twelve years ago in Philadelphia following studies at Temple University. In 1973, he participated in the establishment of the East West Foundation in Boston, and served as Executive Vice-President from 1974–78. During that time, he initiated the annual Conferences on Cancer and Degenerative Illnesses and has written or edited numerous publications on the macrobiotic approach, including *Natural Healing through Macrobiotics* by Michio Kushi and *Macrobiotic Cooking for Everyone*. He has lectured throughout the United States, and in Europe and Japan, and is presently a senior consultant for the East West Foundation and an instructor at the Kushi Institute in Boston.

Frank Kern is a graduate of Virginia Wesleyan College, where he received a B.A. in Psychology in 1971. He did graduate course work in Rehabilitation and Counseling from 1972–74 at the University of North Carolina and Old Dominion University. From 1972–74 he served as the Clinical Services Director of the Tidewater Detention Homes in Virginia Beach, Virginia. He is presently the Assistant Director for the Tidewater Detention Homes and a national, state, and local consultant for behavior modification using diet and nutrition as a primary focus.

Peter Klein, M.D. graduated from LSU Medical School in 1972, and practiced a rotating internship at LAC-USC Medical Center. He conducted his first year psychiatry residency at Mt. Sinai Hospital in Los Angeles from 1973–4, and his second and third year residency at the

UCLA veteran's hospital. He also received a fellowship in child psychology at Reis-Davis-USC Medical Center in 1976–77, and worked with the Los Angeles County Probation Department from 1977–79. He has been engaged in full time private practice since 1980, and is currently the medical director of the Rica Regional Institute for Children and Adolescents in Rockville, Maryland. Dr. Klein has studied and practiced macrobiotics since 1975.

Lawrence H. Kushi received his B.A. from Amherst College in 1978. He is presently a doctoral student in the Department of Nutrition at the Harvard School of Public Health, and is participating with Frank Sacks, M.D. and associates at the Harvard School of Medicine in research dealing with the macrobiotic diet.

Michio Kushi was born in Kokawa, Wakayama Prefecture, Japan in 1926. His early years were devoted to the study of international law at the University of Tokyo, and an active interest in world peace through world federal government in the period following the Second World War. In the course of pursuing these interests, he encountered Yukikazu Sakurazawa (known in the West as George Ohsawa), who had revised and reintroduced the principles of Oriental medicine and philosophy under the name "macrobiotics." Inspired by Mr. Ohsawa's teaching, Mr. Kushi began his lifelong study of the application of traditional understanding to solving the problems of the modern world.

Mr. Kushi came to the United States more than thirty years ago to pursue graduate studies at Columbia University. Since that time he has lectured on Oriental medicine, philosophy, culture and macrobiotics throughout North and South America, Europe and the Far East; he has also given numerous seminars on macrobiotics and Oriental medicine for medical professionals and personal counseling for individuals and families, including many cancer patients. While establishing himself as the world's foremost authority on the macrobiotic approach, he has guided thousands of people to restore their physical, psychological and spiritual health and well-being as a fundamental means of achieving world peace. He has also presented an address to a special White House meeting and two addresses to the delegates of the United Nations on the applications of macrobiotic principles to world problems.

Mr. Kushi is founder and president of the East West Foundation, a federally-approved, non-profit, cultural and educational organization, established in Boston in 1972 to help develop and spread all aspects of the macrobiotic way of life through seminars, publications, research, and other means. He is also the founder of Erewhon, Inc. the leading distributor of natural and macrobiotic foods in North America, and of the monthly *East West Journal* and the quarterly *Order of the Universe* periodicals. In 1978 Mr. and Mrs. Kushi founded the Michio Kushi Institute of Boston, an educational institution for the training of macrobiotic teachers and practitioners, with affiliates in London and Amsterdam; and at the same time, as a further means toward addressing world problems, established the annual Macrobiotic Congresses of North America and Western Europe. A non-profit organization, the Kushi Foundation, was established in 1981 to assist with the coordination of educational and research activities.

Mr. Kushi's published works presently include *Natural Healing through Macrobiotics, The Book of Macrobiotics, The Book of Dō-In, How to See Your Health, Oriental Diagnosis, Visions of a New World: The Era of Humanity*, and the quarterly *Order of the Universe*. Mr. Kushi presently resides in Brookline, Mass., with his wife Aveline and children.

Robert S. Mendelsohn, M.D. has served as Associate Professor, Department of Preventive Medicine, Abraham Lincoln School of Medicine, University of Illinois; Medical Director, American International Hospital, Zion, Illinois; and National Director, Medical Consulation Service, Project Head Start. He is a well-known author, through his nationally syndicated column, *The People's Doctor*, and his recent books, *Confessions of a Medical Heretic* and *Male Practice*. One of the leading medical advocates of the macrobiotic approach, Dr. Mendelsohn had called for the inclusion of courses on macrobiotics and nutrition in medical schools and has authored introductions to several of Mr. Kushi's books. Dr. Mendelsohn presently resides and practices in Evanston, Illinois.

Tom Monte, journalist, and author, has worked as a staff writer for the Center for Science in the Public Interest in Washington, D.C. His story on Dr. Anthony Sattilaro's successful recovery from cancer through macrobiotics, *An M.D. Heals Himself of Cancer*, has appeared in the *East West Journal*, the *Denver Post* and other major newspapers, and the *Saturday Evening Post*. Mr. Monte has served as an Associate Editor for the *East West Journal*, and is the co-authour with Dr. Sattilaro of *Recalled by Life: The Story of a Recovery from Cancer* published by Houghton-Mifflin.

Christiane Northrup, M.D. graduated Phi Beta Kappa from Case Western Reserve University, Cleveland, Ohio in 1971 and from the Dartmouth Medical School in 1975. She has served as Superintendent of Out-Patient Obstetrics and Gynecology at St. Margaret's Hospital in Boston, and as Clinical Assistant Professor of Obstetrics and Gynecology at Tufts Medical School. In January, 1981, she began private practice at the Maine Medical Center in Portland, Maine. Dr. Northrup has appeared regularly at macrobiotic conferences and educational events since 1980.

Hideo Ohmori studied in Japan under George Ohsawa, and has since established himself as the foremost practitioner of macrobiotic healing in Japan. He has successfully treated thousands of patients, including numerous cancer cases, using macrobiotic dietary directions and traditional external treatments. He is presently living and practicing in Tokyo, where he is affiliated with the Nippon Macrobiotic Center.

Norman O. Ralston, D.V.M. is director of the Grove Animal Clinic in Dallas, Texas, where he has successfully pioneered the incorporation of macrobiotic dietary principles and external treatments into his veterinary practice. Dr. Ralston is a frequent participant in macrobiotic conferences and educational programs.

Kristen Schmidt, R.N. received her A.A. Degree at the University of Cincinnati and her R.N. at the University of New Mexico in Albuquerque. From 1974–76, she worked as a staff nurse, specializing in labor and delivery, at Northwestern Memorial Hospital in Chicago. From 1976–80, she was a staff nurse, with a specialty in adolescent psychiatry and labor and delivery, at the University of Cincinnati General Hospital.

Paul Schulman is a health care administrator and consultant. He is the former director of the Lemuel Shattuck Hospital in Boston, where he initiated a macrobiotic meal program, along with programs using acupuncture, yoga, and massage for patients suffering from pain and stress. He has worked at several major medical centers in the United States, including the Mt. Sinai Medical Center, the New York University Medical Center, and the Montefiore Hospital, and is currently an adjunct Assistant Professor at the Tufts Medical School in Boston.

William Tara has been presenting the macrobiotic approach to health through public lectures, seminars for medical professionals and personal counseling throughout Western Europe and the United States for over fifteen years. He is the founder of the Michio Kushi Institute and the Community Health Foundation in London, and is editor of *Oriental Diagnosis* by Michio Kushi. Mr. Tara is currently serving as the Educational Director of the Kushi Institute in Boston.

Index